Glen

I'll Do It Myself

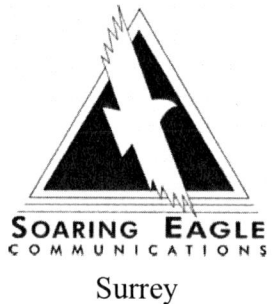

Surrey

I'll Do It Myself
Copyright © 2006 Glenda Watson Hyatt

All rights reserved. No part of this book may be reproduced, stored in a retrieval system, or transmitted, in any form or by any means, without prior written consent of the publisher, except for brief quotations in reviews.

Soaring Eagle Communications
Suite 316, 13910 – 101st Avenue
Surrey, BC Canada V3T 1L6
Website: www.doitmyselfblog.com

Library and Archives Canada Cataloguing in Publication

Hyatt, Glenda Watson, 1966-
    I'll do it myself / Glenda Watson Hyatt.

ISBN 0-9781850-1-3

    1. Hyatt, Glenda Watson, 1966-. 2. Cerebral palsied--British Columbia--Surrey--Biography. I. Title.

RC388.H93A3 2006   362.196'8360092
C2006-906416-4

*To my loving husband Darrell
for his unwavering support and encouragement
in making my dream become reality*

Table of Contents

Introduction	1
In the Beginning	3
Family Life	10
Occasional and Part-Time Thinkers	16
Hospital Stays	20
School Daze	29
Guiding Lights	42
Horsing Around	57
High School	66
Country Life	80
Atop the Hill	92
The Power of One	111
Meet Your Mentor	116
On a Seat Built for Two	123
Wedding Jitters	126
The Eagle Takes Flight	132
From the Heart	144
Baby, Baby, Baby	148
Unenlightened Souls	151
Healing Hands	155
Coming Out of the Silence	166
Epilogue	172

INTRODUCTION

I have dreamt of writing this book, my autobiography, since I was around the age of ten. Egotistical? Perhaps. I see it more as part of my legacy, as my way of passing on the lessons I've learned in hopes of making someone else's life easier, as my way of showing that having cerebral palsy is not a *death* sentence, but rather a *life* sentence.

First, and foremost, I am writing this book for youth and young adults with cerebral palsy and other disabilities to motivate, to inspire and to share how I have navigated life. Sometimes simply reading how someone else handled a particular situation gives the reader the encouragement and ideas for handling a similar situation. Other times knowing others have had similar experiences – to know one is not alone – can be so comforting, and can offer strength and hope.

Secondly, I am also writing this for parents, who, after having their bundle of joy gently placed in their awaiting arms, are given the devastating news their baby has cerebral palsy. In an instant, their hopes and dreams for their child, as well as for their family, are smashed. I hope this book offers a glimmer of hope for these parents, as well as for the siblings, grandparents, aunts and uncles. I want to show that life can still be meaningful, despite cerebral palsy. I hope the book offers parents insights and ideas when raising a child with cp; however, realizing that no two children with cp are the same, there is no guarantee these ideas will be appropriate for every child.

I am also hoping that Human Resources managers, who want to do the right thing by hiring employees with disabilities but still have fears and uncertainties because they don't know anyone with a disability, will experience an increased comfort level being around people with physical disabilities and will venture into the pool of underutilized skills, talents and knowledge.

This book is also for individuals who enjoy reading about the lives of others in order to gain a new understanding of other people or to gain a new perspective or insight into their own life.

Lastly, I hope the book will enable doctors and medical professionals to see beyond the diagnosis, the prognosis and the *can'ts*, and see the patient as a person filled with capabilities, potential and desires. However, that may be expecting far too much from only one book!

Thank you for reading and for sharing in my dream.

In the Beginning

I entered this world one Friday morning in early November, 1966, in Vancouver, British Columbia. A light dusting of snow covered the ground. Mom said the North Shore Mountains looked like upside down pink ice cream cones as the sun rose outside her hospital room window.

My parents were living in Nanaimo on Vancouver Island, but Mom's doctor wanted her to give birth at Grace Hospital in Vancouver. Nanaimo did have a hospital, but according to Mom's doctor, it was merely a first aid post in a hospital building. Any serious cases were airlifted to Victoria or Vancouver. Perhaps it was doctor's intuition that wanted her at the best maternity hospital in the province at that time.

Mom travelled over to Vancouver in mid-October to stay with her parents, my Nana and Papa, while Dad stayed in Nanaimo to work. Mom and Nana enjoyed those couple of weeks before my birth, shopping for baby things at Woodward's $1.49 Day. If Mom's relationship with Nana was anything like my relationship with Mom, I have no doubt that they had silly fun and good laughs during those two weeks.

Mom had a normal pregnancy, and everything was fine up until my actual arrival. Then the situation became somewhat scary and uncertain. Mom had a reaction to the Xylocaine epidural and went into convulsions. The doctor had to pull me out with forceps, which meant I didn't have time to read the instructions on my way down the chute. I missed the fine print on needing to breathe immediately.

One doctor worked on reviving Mom, while another one worked on saving me. Luckily, a pediatrician specialist was just leaving the hospital and was called back to try to get me breathing. Perhaps it wasn't a coincidence that the specialist was there at that particular moment. He was probably one of the angels sent to save me that day. It was touch and go for a while. Dad nearly lost both of us.

I definitely would not have held my breath for six minutes had I known what hassles it would cause for the rest of my life. Talk about learning from experience. You would think the first lesson for a newborn would be somewhat easier!

I was blue for a good part of my first day and was placed in the "no touch zone" as the intensive care nursery was called in those days. Only the doctors and nurses were allowed to touch me. Mom could only stand at the window and watch me. Apparently she would not go back to her room until she saw me move. She prayed hard that day that I would live. Live I did!

By the time Dad arrived from Nanaimo some time that weekend, I was *baby girl pink*. However, I was kept in the "no touch zone" for seven days. On the fourth day, Mom was finally allowed to hold and to nurse me. Holding me took some effort as I was like a limp rag doll. I had absolutely no muscle tone. Nursing was also a struggle as I had problems sucking; feeding me took quite a while.

Being small and white, Mom wanted to name me Edelweiss, a reference from her all-time favourite movie *Sound of Music*. But she realized Edelweiss Watson did not sound quite right, so my parents settled on the name Glenda. In later years this decision proved to be a slight curse for me as 'G' is difficult for me to pronounce. And, for some unknown reason, people insist on asking "What is your name?" upon meeting for the first time. Is it Linda? Brenda? Heidi? Conversations do not get off to a good start when we can't even get my name right. It doesn't really matter what people call me as long as they do it with respect.

Although the long-term implications were still unknown, I had apparent problems. Adding to the complications, Mom developed pneumonia as a result of swallowing fluids into her lungs while she was having convulsions. Once we were both relatively stable, we were released from the hospital ten days after my birth. We went home to Nana's and Papa's house because the doctors wanted us to remain in Vancouver for a couple weeks to make sure I kept sucking properly. The extended stay also provided Mom with some help as she recovered from her pneumonia. Nana enjoyed digging through her old trunk for a few sweaters and blankets she had saved from when Mom was a baby.

Finally, at the end of November, nearly a month after my birth, Mom was allowed to take me home to Nanaimo. Without an *official* diagnosis or prognosis, the doctor simply said, "Take her home and love her." Papa drove us to the Canadian Pacific Railway (CPR) ferry terminal, where he worked, and Mom carried me onboard in the white wicker bassinette. Dad anxiously picked us up on the other side in Nanaimo.

Mom quickly found a doctor for me in Nanaimo. However, being the first baby with my symptoms that he had ever encountered beyond textbooks in medical school, although the diagnosis *cerebral palsy* had yet to be uttered out loud, he recommended that Mom continue to have my check ups in Vancouver. Mom and I rode on the CPR ferry Princess Marguerite, which Papa helped maintain, many times as we travelled back and forth between Nanaimo and Vancouver for my doctor appointments.

Nanaimo's Public Health Nurse came to check on me, as she did with all new babies, and asked how Mom was washing my diapers (this was long before disposable ones). Since my parents did not have a washer or dryer and could not afford to go to the laundromat, Mom explained how she washed the diapers in bleach water in the bathtub, boiled them in a pot on the stove and then hung them to dry in what was the laundry room (minus the washer and dryer). The nurse was absolutely mortified! She said Mom simply could not do it that way. Mom was thinking, *Why not? I don't use the soup pot; I use another pot. At least I don't have to chop wood first for a fire like they did in the 'old days'!* Mom doesn't recall ever hearing from that nurse again. Sometimes one must make do with what one has, and Mom was doing just that!

It was quite some time before I was officially diagnosed with cerebral palsy, or more accurately, cerebral palsy athetoid quadriplegia. The lack of oxygen had caused permanent brain damage, resulting in a lack of muscle control and coordination. My physical movements are jerky and involuntary; one body part or another is in constant motion. My left hand has some function, while my right hand is generally in a tightly clenched fist. I can't walk without support, and my speech is difficult to understand. Finally, my head control is tenuous, and swallowing takes a conscious effort.

At six months of age, one doctor in Vancouver offered the opinion that I was mentally retarded and that I should be institutionalized. That would have meant a life with little or no contact with my family or the outside world. I would have received minimal education, living a life without hope or opportunity. Thankfully, my parents had their own unflattering opinion of that medical professional and did not follow his bleak recommendation.

My first summer found me off to church camp. Nothing like an early start! Mom had been to Camp Artaban as a teen, and then as a leader and a staff member. Artaban, which is still operated by the Anglican Church today, is a rustic waterfront camp located on Gambier Island in Howe Sound, about 20 miles by water from Vancouver. Mom was slated to be on staff for one or two of the two-week camps that summer. Since Dad could not afford to take time off work to care for a ten-month-old baby, Mom simply took me to camp with her. She packed my clothes, cloth diapers and baby food in the bottom of a steamer trunk. The top tray was my camp bed! Diapers were washed in an agitating washtub and hand-cranked wringer and hung on the line to dry.

The inscription on the handwritten camp completion certificate, dated August 10, 1967, says:

Glenda is our mascot,

She is our pride and joy,

We all love her an awful lot

Because she's not a boy.

Obviously, I was not an imposition at camp. There was no need to constantly watch me or to run after me, as is the case with most toddlers, because I stayed put, perfectly content to sit propped up in my stroller and watch the activities of the campers.

The end of summer found us moving back to Vancouver as Dad had a new job as a salesman with a construction news service. We stayed with Nana and Papa again until my parents found a house to buy. Mom's sister Fern was still living at home, too, so it was quite cozy with the six of us in a small, two-bedroom house. Apparently, I wasn't too happy with a houseful of people. I had an overactive startle reflex, a quirk of cp that I have never outgrown, that caused me to jump any time someone moved or talked. I still tend to jump out of my chair when someone comes up behind me or speaks loudly, particularly when I am tired or stressed. It is simply one of those things I can't really control, no matter how hard I try. That is life with cp.

After much searching, Mom and Dad found a house out *in the sticks* that they could afford – a six-month-old house in Port Coquitlam, then considered a fair distance from Vancouver; now, with urban sprawl, it is a mere suburb. Papa went down in his basement and brought back up a tobacco can with $500, an extraordinary amount of money in those days. That was our down payment! The house had a wringer washing machine and a clothesline, luxuries compared to the home in Nanaimo. We were there for nearly one year until the monthly mortgage payment increased by five dollars, forcing my parents to sell. Although it does not sound like a substantial increase by today's standards, in those days, milk was 29¢ per quart, cigarettes were 47¢ a pack, and gas was a measly 42¢ per gallon!

Our family moved into a garden apartment in Burnaby, next door to Vancouver; not far from Nana's and Papa's house. We lived there for a few years, and this is the first home I vaguely remember. I remember riding my plastic tractor. I couldn't use the squeaky foot pedals to propel it because I did not have the coordination, so I pushed it with my feet on the ground. It worked! One day, the apartment superintendent had tired of listening to the noisy foot pedals. He brought out a hacksaw and cut them off! I didn't mind as they were in my way anyway. We were both happy!

Around that time, I started my school career at the *Yellow Submarine*, a special needs preschool at the University of British Columbia. One day, the psychologist, Dr. Kendall, came by to test if anything was going on in my damaged brain.

At that point in my life, my speech was very limited, consisting primarily of initial consonants and sounds. Going through the Peabody Vocabulary Picture Test, I uttered one response that he simply could not understand. Finally, in complete desperation, he called in Mom, who was observing from behind the *magic mirror* (actually a one-way window), to decipher what I was saying. *Roo roo.* The two of them gazed at the picture of a chicken. *Roo roo.* Suddenly it dawned on Mom. She asked, "Glenda, do you mean rooster?" Yes! The picture was obviously a rooster as it had a big, red comb. The experts expected me to offer the accepted response – chicken. Who was called mentally retarded?

Dr. Kendall reported that I was *bright* and showed potential. After all, I knew the difference between a chicken and a rooster before the age of three. Even with this encouraging report from the psychologist, I would be required to prove my capabilities and potential countless times throughout my life as so many people don't see beyond the cerebral palsy to see me.

FAMILY LIFE

Following the only advice given by the doctor after my birth, my parents did take me home and love me. In the late 1960s, support was non-existent for parents who had children with special needs. My parents were left to figure out things on their own; they did the best they knew how at the time. Who could ask for more?

Mom was still completing her degree in education, with a specialty in Special Education – lucky me! Thus she had access to the medical library at the University of British Columbia, where she spent time reading about cerebral palsy and searching for answers to questions that could not yet be answered by the doctors.

Much of the time my parents muddled along, trying different approaches until they found one that worked. In the early years, feeding was definitely a major issue. Placed in the plastic cuddle seat on the table, I had a short attention span when it came to eating pabulum and other mushy baby food. I was either more interested in what was happening around me, or I was bored because it took so long to finish a meal. Dad learned to keep my attention while feeding me by sticking my favourite rattle, which had a suction cup, on his forehead. I doubt that idea was in a Special Ed textbook but rather an idea attempted out of sheer desperation!

Next was the high chair with a towel tied around my middle to hold me up. One time when Dad was feeding me, I picked up the spoon and threw it on the floor. Dad firmly said "No", picked it up and placed it back on the tray. I did it again. Dad repeated his stern no. I did it again and, perhaps, again. Dad lightly smacked my hand. I cried. Dad went into his bedroom and cried. The incident taught both Daddy and his little girl that having cerebral palsy did not preclude me from discipline. That may have been the first incident of discipline, but it was definitely not the last!

As I grew and gained some hand control to do more than throw the spoon on the floor, I was able to feed myself, more or less. It was a slow process. I was nearly always left sitting alone at the table as I finished my supper. Some nights I exerted more energy than I gained by eating. It's no wonder I was so skinny. The process wasn't pretty, especially when I was tired, causing my involuntary movements to be even less controllable. Those mealtimes often resulted in a battle and tears at the dinner table. Perhaps this is why I'm still uncomfortable eating around others not close to me and try almost anything to avoid it.

When I graduated from my crib (and steamer trunk) to my first bed, the bed was actually a mattress on the floor. At that time I was getting around by crawling on my hands and knees. By having my bed directly on the floor, I was able to crawl in and out of bed myself. Independence was important, even at a young age.

When we moved from the small, two-bedroom garden apartment to the larger townhouse in Surrey, I had my own bedroom with space for an actual bed. I was given the one Mom had as a child. To ensure the bed was still low enough for me to climb into by myself, Dad cut a sheet of plywood to lay across the bedrails, with the foam mattress on top. Who needs a box spring!

Along the way, my parents blessed me with three brothers: Kevin, Neal and Ian. The third time around I really wanted a baby sister. Dad claims that when he woke me up and informed me that I had another brother, I punched my pillow. However, my disappointment quickly disappeared, and I loved my newest brother Ian, who remains my *baby* brother to this day, regardless of our ages. I simply must remember not to call him that when he is standing too close!

Although brothers could be pretty *weird* and *annoying* creatures at times, none of them had any physical problems like mine. I recall one time playing with them all in my bedroom and Neal, who was five or six years old, remarked, "When you become a boy, you will walk, too." His comment made perfect sense in a sweet, innocent sort of way, although I am not quite sure how he rationalized the fact that Mom could walk. Perhaps in his mind she was a mommy, not a girl! It's fascinating how young minds work.

The early years were happy times for us as we did much together as a family. In the late spring and summer months, we went camping in our tent trailer. On one weekend camping trip, we had barely finished eating, and I was still sitting in my wheelchair at one end of the picnic table with my tray attached to my wheelchair. A cheeky squirrel scampered on to the table in search of scraps. He neared my end of the table. I sat still, which is not an easy task with athetoid cp. He ventured onto the corner of my tray long enough to leave his footprints on my white tray. I was so excited that I wanted to take the tray to school on Monday morning for Show n Tell. Mom witnessed the whole encounter, and I wouldn't let her wipe off the tray for the rest of the weekend.

Monday morning Mom dropped me off in my classroom, putting the tray in the corner with the other ones, and then walked down the hall to her room as she was a Special Education teacher in the same school. The aide came in and, noticing the "dirt" on my tray, dutifully took it to the sink to wash it off. Very disappointed, I watched as my Show n Tell was washed down the sink. I was too afraid to say anything because she probably wouldn't understand me; after all, I'm *non-verbal*.

In the winter, we went snowshoeing. Dad rigged up a child's wooden sleigh for me. Wrapped in a Teflon rescue blanket, I stayed fairly warm during family outings. One time, Dad jumped in a snow bank, creating a hole waist high, and stood me in it. It was better than any wooden standing table used to keep me in an upright position. On that particular outing, as we trudged through the snow, Neal was quite concerned that we were trampling on "baby trees". Dad tried explaining that, because the snow was so deep, those were actually the tops of trees, but I'm not sure if Neal believed him. Mom made spaghetti for lunch on the propane camp stove, using melted snow to boil the noodles. Those were happy family times!

The six of us were actively involved in the Guiding and Scouting movements, which were part of our way of life rather than only a meeting we attended once a week. Our lives were busy with newspaper drives, outings, weekend camps, and projects for badges.

Then there was the Watson menagerie – gerbils, birds, dogs, cats, guinea pigs, rabbits, and fish. Our family included every type of pet, except a horse, at one time or another. At one point we bred Shelties, and Dad built a large whelping pen in our kitchen/eating area. I would get down on the floor, open the pen door, sit in the doorway and play with the puppies. At times it was so much easier to be with animals than with people as the animals didn't care about my unclear speech or my jerky movements. Selling a puppy felt like selling a friend – heartbreaking.

Despite money being tight, we always had what we truly needed. Mom did the best with what food we had, although we still tease her about the disastrous meal she concocted when all that was left in the cupboard was sauerkraut, bacon, and mushroom soup. We enjoyed homemade muffins, cookies, bannock, and ground beef cooked in 1001 ways. We definitely did not starve; however, getting to the food before my brothers ate it all was a challenge.

In the mid 1980s, during the 18% mortgage years, the six of us each drew the name of the family member for whom we would buy a Christmas present. Of course, we had a spending limit, which made it challenging to find the perfect gift. Figuring out which name each person had drawn was part of the fun.

One Saturday morning in late November, Kevin asked Mom to drive him to the shopping mall because he had an idea for his gift, and it was on sale that day. Mom drove him to the mall and waited for him at a specified location. Shortly afterwards, Kevin returned with a small box, slightly upset: "Mom, there was tax! I need a few more cents." Mom gave him the required change and held the box as he raced back to the store. The box meowed!

The Friday evening before, I had been to the mall and had seen this cute orange and white kitty with a tiny smudge of black in the pet store. I mentioned it at the dinner table that night, emphasizing how she was almost the colour of my red hair. Earlier that year my Siamese-Persian kitty Imp died mysteriously, and in typical parent style, Mom had consoled me by saying I could get another kitty *one day*. I don't think Mom had planned on *one day* being quite that moment, but she didn't have the heart to tell Kevin that he couldn't buy his sister a kitty – one that she would love instantly – for Christmas. Besides, it was within the set spending limit, except for the tax. Amber joined the family.

Occasional and Part-Time Thinkers

Beginning around the time of the *Yellow Submarine* and lasting for roughly a decade, I had therapy – physio, occupational and speech – several times each week. This was necessary to improve balance, muscle coordination and verbal communication. While therapy was necessary, it was seldom fun; like taking foul-tasting medicine.

Physio and occupational therapy involved monotonous tasks, such as repeatedly grasping beanbags and putting them in muffin tins, climbing up a few stairs to simply reach a brick wall, and being rolled around on a large, inflated ball or tube. This was all done stripped to my underwear. When I became older, I was permitted to wear shorts and a top.

Speech therapy seemed rather bizarre to me. The therapist sat on a floor mat with me lying on my back between her outstretched legs. My legs wrapped around her waist, and her stinky toes were in close proximity to my nose. She then proceeded to stick her fingers in my mouth to wiggle my lips, supposedly to loosen them. She alternated between using her fingers and ice cubes. When the speaking segment of the therapy began, she pushed on my chest in attempts to improve my breathing capacity. After years of this hefty woman pushing down on my chest, I am convinced that was why I was such a late bloomer.

As I laid on my back staring at the ceiling tiles, I was puzzled. *What was I supposed to do when I met people in the real world? Lay down on my back, on the floor, before speaking to them?* I envisioned myself sprawled out on the ground when meeting a friend at the shopping mall or grocery store. This was not a dignified thought. Not surprisingly, pillow talk is some of my clearest speech!

In most cases, my therapists were not the brightest individuals. One day I came home from Kindergarten, nearly in tears. *Mommy, my knees hurt.* She sat me down and looked at my long-legged braces. The occupational therapist (OT) had put them on the wrong legs! Wearing shoes on the wrong feet causes some discomfort, but wearing heavy, metal braces on the wrong legs hurts. No doubt, I knew he was putting the wrong brace on the wrong leg. However, being *nonverbal*, I likely kept quiet, something I often did, because I thought he wouldn't understand what I was saying, and I didn't want to create a big hassle as he tried to decipher what I was telling him. After all, only people close to me understood *Glenda-ish*.

Feeding myself was always a struggle, and oftentimes ended in a battle and tears. To this day I don't mind eating alone and, at times, would actually prefer it. The OT suggested that bending a spoon ninety degrees may make it easier for me to get the spoon into my mouth, a great idea. The next week, I took the spoon in my left hand, my only somewhat functional hand, and was all set to . . . feed the OT. He had bent the spoon the wrong way! Thankfully, it was not one of Mom's good spoons.

In a similar attempt, he thought a swivel spoon might do the trick. This spoon had a large, plastic handle to grip and a spoon bowl turned ninety degrees, in the correct direction, which actually swiveled. Well, between my jerky, uncoordinated movements and this spoon swinging back and forth, the peas ended up across the room! I continued using a plain, unaltered spoon.

As I started elementary school, it was apparent that an electric typewriter would be useful. My parents bought a Smith Corona typewriter for me to use at home. The OT suggested that a keyguard may prevent me from hitting multiple keys at once, and he offered to make it himself. Super. Months later he finished drilling the holes in a piece of Plexiglas. When installing the handmade keyguard onto the typewriter, it was discovered that there were more holes than keys! Another OT solution was tossed on the junk heap. Luckily, Smith Corona also made keyguards.

Because I was such a cheerful and cooperative client, I was always given to the newest therapists, probably to break them in easily. It seemed like I would only get one "trained" when a new one would join the Treatment Centre's staff, and I had to start over yet again. Sometimes it doesn't pay to be cooperative.

When I was ten or eleven, I had one OT who had me actually make things. She took me into the workshop and allowed me to use some of the tools. That was cool! I remember making a wooden doll bed. I even painted it, too. Then one day she told Mom, "Glenda figures out how to do things on her own, in her own way. She doesn't need me. We are wasting her time here." I finally had a therapist who made sense and actually understood me, and I had to let her go.

If memory serves me correctly, speech therapy ended around the same time. After the speech therapist with stinky toes, I had one for a brief time who had me sit upright for the entire session. What a concept! One of the most sensible things we did was make an alphabet card, small enough to carry with me, which I could use when people didn't understand what I was saying. I simply spelled out the word on the card. Sometimes the low-tech solution works the best, and I've had many variations of that card through the years.

Physio therapy came to an end sometime during Grade 8. At this point, physio was mainly to maintain muscle tone and flexibility, which I could now do on my own. Besides, I was getting too big for the current physiotherapist. Mom had to come into the room for specific exercises to spot me, which meant no one was watching my three brothers as they terrorized the lobby area. Had a big, hunky ex-football player-turned-physio been available, I may have been more interested in continuing physio. But, since there was not, I wasn't upset when we decided to discontinue physio. Finally, I was free from that yucky medicine!

Years later, as a wheelchair technician worked on my husband's wheelchair, he commented on some of the "brilliant" adaptations OTs and PTs had him make to chairs. He then revealed that OT stood for Occasional Thinker and PT meant Part-time Thinker. It all made sense now.

Hospital Stays

Having cerebral palsy meant corrective surgeries were inevitable, at least in the late 1960s and 70s, in order to maximize potential mobility and functionality. I was four years old when I had my first surgery, a procedure to release my hamstrings behind my knees and my abductors in my inner thighs to increase flexibility and mobility of my legs.

Prior to the surgery, Dr. Bell placed me in traction in an attempt to stretch and loosen my muscles. While in traction with my feet attached to weights hanging over the end of the hospital crib, I could not get out of bed for three weeks. Try keeping an energetic four-year-old quiet and entertained while confined to bed for weeks, especially in the days before VCRs and computer games. I spent hours with my Etch n Sketch.

I don't recall how I acquired her, but I also had my hospital dollie. She was only three or four inches tall, and she fit in my fisted left hand. Coincidentally, she had long red hair. I kept her with me all the time and was so upset when she was tucked into the bedside drawer as they wheeled me to the operating room. She accompanied me on each subsequent hospital stay.

Adding to the unpleasant nature of my first hospital stay, there was no way I could wear underwear with my feet tied up in the air. After being toilet trained for a couple of years, I was put back in diapers. And, when the staff had to place a cold, uncomfortable bedpan under me, I was not impressed. Worst of all, my parents were not allowed to stay with me in the hospital. When Mom and Dad had to leave at the end of visiting hours, there were tears on both sides of the door. I still dread saying good-bye to this day.

Finally, the surgery was performed. I came out of the operating room in a hip spica cast that extended from my ankles to my armpits, with my legs spread wide apart. Looking like an upside-down Y, I was completely immobilized and dependent – not fun, to say the least! I would stay like that for six months.

Shortly after the surgery, I was not sent home. Instead, I was sent to recuperate at Sunny Hill Hospital, which was like a rehab centre for children. For some children with physical disabilities who were institutionalized or abandoned by their parents, Sunny Hill was home. Doctors were in charge, and my parents had little say.

Like clockwork, my parents and two brothers (Ian was not yet born) came to visit me daily. Naturally, there were tears when they left because I couldn't go home with them, and I didn't like being left alone. The hospital was a frightening place for a small, vulnerable child, especially when the staff and nurses couldn't understand me. They generally didn't talk to me or tell me what they were about to do to me.

The social worker strongly recommended to Mom that they not visit me because I became so upset when they left. Mom refused. I was part of the family, and they would come daily. The worker then suggested that they only come Sundays, which was the official family day. Mom repeated her statement about coming daily. In one last attempt to reduce the number of crying children, the worker offered that I have only two visitors per day. Mom once again held her position, refusing to back down. We did things as a family – a whole family. They would all come to see me each day. This was one area where, as a parent, she had some control. She wasn't about to abandon me, even short-term, in such a place. The worker finally conceded.

Eventually, I was allowed to go home on weekends. As the doctor signed my release for my first weekend home, he ordered my parents to ensure that I had a quiet weekend. "Yes, Doctor. No problem," they assured him. Bright and early Saturday morning, we lined up for the Shriners' Parade. Mom and Dad propped me, in my Y-shaped cast, against the curb so that I could see everything. One Shriner passed by and tucked a $5 bill in my hand. Awhile later, another Shriner tucked a $5 bill in my other fisted hand "so that I was balanced." The clowns, the noise, and the action combined were more excitement than I had experienced in several months.

With the parade over and our car packed, we then went camping with friends. A hike was part of the plan and not to exclude me from the group, Dad and Uncle Jim carried me in my heavy body cast the entire way. Upon returning to our campsite, we discovered a Styrofoam cooler does not withstand bears. Oh, what a mess! And, probably not quite what the doctor had meant by a quiet weekend! But, oh what fun!

Other weekends weren't as wild. Eventually my cast was split into two – a front and a back – so that I could get out for brief periods. Mom would sit on the floor with me sitting between her outstretched legs. With a child's magnet board over my lap to keep my legs straight, we read stories, assembled jigsaw puzzles or played games, enjoying quality time together like any mother and child.

On Monday morning, I would tearfully return to Sunny Hill. It seemed like we were served scrambled eggs and green beans for supper day after day. After six months of scrambled eggs and green beans, I could hardly stomach either one again! To make matters even worse, if a nurse wasn't available or if a parent wasn't present at an occasional meal time, I was placed on my board with casters. A dish was put on the floor in front of me, and I had to eat off the floor like a dog. This was a totally humiliating and degrading experience for a child.

Decades later, I attended a committee meeting at Sunny Hill, and I suffered my first and only panic attack. My stomach was in knots and breathing was difficult. I wanted to run. After ten minutes I was able to cross the street and to enter the place that had left an indelible mark on my memory. My stay as a child may have been necessary, but it wasn't pleasant. I did not linger after that meeting, and the next time the committee met at Sunny Hill, I was *regrettably* busy.

Once I was finished with the cast, I returned to Sunny Hill as a patient one last time to get my first wheelchair. As a four-year-old, I didn't appreciate the significance of what a wheelchair symbolized – that I was disabled, different, less of a person in the eyes of some; that walking, a capability unfathomably valued by society, would not be my primary means of mobility; that it would give complete strangers license to stare, to pity, and for parents to pull their children away from me for fear that I was contagious. I was only excited because it was red – my favourite colour! What else could be more important in my young mind?

My second surgery entailed cutting my heel cords to release the tightness. Except for the bedpans, yucky red pre-op medicine, and being wheeled in my bed down endless corridors to the operating room, I don't remember much about that hospital stay. I do remember kicking my feet in the air as Mom and Dad walked into the ward after the surgery. I was so excited and relieved that I only had to wear small bootie casts, a dramatic difference from my first cast.

I don't recall being in the hospital for too long after the surgery, and I went straight home upon release – not to Sunny Hill, thank goodness! However, I do remember my parents bringing in our young Sheltie dog Bonnie to see me. This was long before the benefits of pet therapy were medically known, so Mom and Dad had to do quite a song and dance to receive permission to take a dog into the sterile hospital. It definitely brightened my day!

Over the next few years, my only hospital stays were for dental work. Because of my lack of mouth control, I couldn't have dental work – beyond a basic cleaning – done in the dentist chair. Instead, I spent a night in the hospital until they came up with the day surgery option. I never completely understood those days. Mom woke me up early to get to the hospital on time. Then I was given that yucky, red sedation medicine, which made my eyes water. I would cough and choke and get emotional and teary. Once in the O.R., they would cover my face with the black rubber gas mask – the mere thought of it makes me cringe and feel claustrophobic. When the work was done and I was in recovery, a nurse would wake me up and ask me my name. I simply pointed to my ID bracelet, thinking: *Would you guys make up your minds, please? Do you want me awake or asleep? I'm asleep now, so leave me be.*

I still dread each trip to the hospital, no matter how brief. To this day I turn green, literally, upon entering a hospital for any reason, even when visiting a friend on the maternity ward.

The third surgery recommended by my pediatric orthopedic surgeon was a triple arthrodesis – try saying that with *Glenda-ish* – to stabilize my ankles. They were beginning to turn over, causing me to walk on the side of them. Without the surgery, this condition would worsen, making walking even a few steps both harmful and painful. With the surgery, I might graduate from long-legged braces to those only below the knee. Because I was ten years old, Mom and Dad left the decision completely up to me. They felt it was my body and my choice, and they said they would support my decision either way. What a decision for a kid to make! What a responsibility!

Dr. Bell explained the procedure to me in very simple terms. He would rearrange the bones in my ankles and then wire them together until they fused. This might limit the range of motion in my foot, but it would prevent the ankle from turning further on its side. Mom took me to the hospital to visit a classmate who had received the same surgery so that I could get first-hand insight into what the surgery was really like and how it felt afterwards. I weighed my fear of hospitals against the potential benefits and, after much anxiety-ridden deliberation and many tears, I took a big gulp and decided to take the gamble to have the surgery. A date was set for late in the summer before Grade 6.

My left ankle was operated on first, followed by my right ankle a few days later. The pain was excruciating! Every time I twitched a muscle, which was nearly constantly with athetoid cp, it felt like I re-sprained both ankles. And the more it hurt, the tighter my muscles became, which made it hurt even more! It was a vicious circle! Telling me to relax didn't help much either. I was given various medications to relieve the pain, but the only one that worked moderately well was Demerol. I received injections in my thighs every four hours. Even then I asked for the next injection before the third hour ended. Imagine a kid asking for needles! My thighs soon looked like pin cushions. On one occasion the needle stuck in my leg as my muscle contracted, which scared the nurse. I'm not sure why it made her so nervous; it was stuck in MY leg!

Because of the pain issue, I was in the hospital much longer than expected. I missed the beginning of the school year, which didn't help my morale because I loved school. The hospital teacher kept coming around, asking if I wanted to have any lessons yet. Although she meant well and was simply doing her job, I found this very annoying. I was in too much pain to focus on mixed fractions; in fact, I wasn't in the mood to do anything more strenuous than watching television. As I was about ready to throw a bedpan at the woman on her next attempt to ask me if I was ready, Mom strongly recommended to the nurses that they not allow the teacher to bother me again.

The extended hospital stay took its toll on my family as they tried juggling work, school, my brothers' Scouting activities and visiting me a few times daily. After teaching all day, Mom spent hours at my bedside, knitting as I cycled through pain and sleep. Dad came in the mornings to help me with breakfast as well as lunch when he could get away from work. My brothers came in the evening, however seeing their sister in so much pain for an extended period began negatively affecting them. My middle brother Neal, the somewhat quiet one and in Grade 3 at the time, drew a picture that alarmed the teacher enough to call my Mom. The picture depicted a doctor in a wheelchair, being pushed towards the edge of a cliff. That was his opinion of the doctor who hurt his sister.

For my long overdue release, our proxy grandma Nana embroidered purple flowers on socks large enough to wear over my casts. It was nearly fall, but it was still a beautiful sunny day. I remember all of us sitting around the family table, eating *well-done* grilled cheese sandwiches. I looked outside our big dining room window and saw two raccoons up in the cedar tree, watching us eat our lunch. Watching them watch us made me laugh, something I hadn't done in a long time. It was good to be home.

One morning as Mom was lifting me out of bed, trying carefully not to bang my two casts together, she tore all the ligaments in her back. She was told not to lift. Who was going to take me to the bathroom? The tooth fairy? Once again the family routine was forced to change. Dad came home from work when he could during the day to take me to the bathroom and to check on Mom, who spent whatever time she could resting in a chaise lounge in the family room. He also took care of the vacuuming and other heavy housework.

Still in my casts, I went back to school and Brownies. Meanwhile, Mom spent her days at physio and in the pool, accompanied by my little brother Ian, who was not school-aged yet. Her recovery was slow and painful.

Finally it was time for my casts to be removed. Because the wires, which were holding my bones together, had to be pulled out, I had to be put to sleep yet again. This required another night or two in the hospital, and I was not thrilled. To add insult to injury, the only bed available was on the infants' ward. I reached my breaking point and I started crying uncontrollably. Mom walked into the room and said, in her no-nonsense manner, "Shh, you are making more noise than the babies." I turned my head towards Dad, who was sitting by my bedside, and said, in between sobbing, "I give up. I don't want to do this any more." That was one of the three times in my life that I remember tears in his eyes. Those words were never uttered in our house; it was always "I will try."

The opportunity arose for the family to go to Hawaii for ten days in mid-December. After the rough fall, my parents felt some fun in the sun would be good for the entire family. We had a great time eating pineapple spears with juice running down our arms, seeing bananas actually growing on trees, and watching a whole pig being cooked in a pit at an authentic luau. The warmth, the scents, and the sights are all fond memories from that trip.

We returned home in time for the last day of school before Christmas holidays. We then traded our summer clothes for winter ones and headed for Forbidden Plateau on Vancouver Island. Auntie Fern and Uncle Ed were managing the ski lodge at that time, and as it was going to be closed over the holidays, we all – including Uncle's parents and our baby cousin Craig – went up for Christmas. We had free run of the rustic lodge atop the ski hill. Uncle Ed was recovering from a serious volleyball mishap, so it was a good way to end a painful and stressful year. It was the best Christmas we ever had as a family!

SCHOOL DAZE

The summer of 1972 saw Mom, myself in a wheelchair, Kevin wearing a child's harness with reins and Neal in a backpack carrier boarding a plane to Scotland for six weeks. (Ian was not yet in the picture, which was probably a good thing as Mom was out of hands!) Dad joined us a few weeks later as he only had three weeks of holidays.

We travelled over to visit with Auntie Fern and Uncle Ed in Edinburgh, where Uncle was working at the time. Prior to our trip, Uncle had sent me a children's picture book of Edinburgh. His plan was to take a photo of me at each one of the landmarks and then affix the photo beside the appropriate picture in the book. One morning, Uncle hollered to Mom, "I'm taking Glenda for the day," as we were headed out the door. Mildly concerned, Mom hollered back, "What if she needs to go to the bathroom?" "Then I'll take her," he responded. Nothing unsavory was intended. That is simply life with cp: sometimes other people must assist with personal needs.

Looking back at those photos, which have since faded with time, I'm not sure how Uncle got the shots, especially one of me leaning in a pub doorway. He must have propped me up and then run like hell down the street to take the picture before either I fell or someone opened the door and I fell.

I vaguely remember exploring underground tunnels at St. Andrews Castle. When the tunnel became too narrow for my borrowed wheelchair, Dad and Uncle took turns carrying me, until it became too narrow for the two of us. For the most part, I wasn't held back from experiencing life simply because I have a so-called disability.

I then began Grade 1 in my purple heather sweater and purple plaid kilt. I was one bonnie lass!

School was an older building; actually, it consisted of two buildings and a portable. The main building had four or five classrooms for the primary grades, the staff room, changing room and the principal's office. The older kids were upstairs in the other building, accessible by a long, steep ramp.

As this was before *integration* and *mainstreaming* had been invented, all the Special Ed students went to this school, which was actually an annex of a larger school, several blocks away. This was definitely segregation. But, at that age, I didn't know any differently. I was excited to be starting school with my new notebooks, crayons and lefty scissors. And, I do remember hating missing school when I was sick. It was so boring to stay home.

Being *non-verbal*, my teacher Mrs. Rutherford was concerned that she wouldn't hear me when I needed help, so she gave me two small brass bells – I think they were her mom's dinner bells – to ring to get her attention. It was soon discovered that the bells weren't necessary as I was verbal enough to catch her attention when needed.

Because getting to the chalkboard was difficult for most of us once we were placed in our seats, we each had an 18-inch square piece of chalkboard at our desks for practicing our printing. It was also easier to work on a horizontal surface rather than a vertical one. Initially, my printing was wobbly scribbles. With practice and extreme concentration, I controlled my jerky movements enough to make my letters almost legible more of the time. I also kept a chalk eraser handy, though inadvertently an uncontrollable movement erased a *good* letter. In frustration, I did the letter again.

Although learning to print, and then to write, were important steps in learning to read, it was evident that printing would not be efficient. It took too much energy and was too time-consuming to keep up with my work, and that would only worsen through the grades. Learning to use a typewriter was a necessity.

An electric Smith Corona typewriter was placed at the back of the room, which a few of us shared. When it was time to do typewriter work, Mrs. Rutherford dragged me in my desk chair over to the typewriter table and then dragged me back to my desk when I was done. Then it was the next student's turn. A while later, perhaps once funding became available, we each had a typewriter at a second desk beside us. We simply dragged the typewriter back and forth as we needed it. It was much easier, especially on Mrs. Rutherford's back.

As I have only one somewhat functioning hand, I only typed with one hand, my left hand. While typing, I steadied my hand on the typewriter *hood* to give myself some control over the spastic movements and used my thumb to hit the keys, causing my wrist to be in a dropped-wrist position. This concerned the adults, particularly the physio and OT. Although this was decades before repetitive strain injury and carpal tunnel syndrome had been invented, they were concerned that the dropped-wrist position would cause damage over the long-term.

They decided a splint with a stick to hit the keys was needed to keep my wrist in a good position. With this contraption snuggly Velcro strapped to my arm, I was expected to have enough arm control to steady my hand mid-air, without resting it on anything, and to accurately hit the keys. And this was less frustrating than printing with a pencil? After a few days, the splint ended up in the back of my desk drawer, and I resumed typing with my left thumb, my hand in its compromising position. I type the same way today, as nothing else feels as natural. For a non-verbal individual who relies on written communication, my left thumb is my most valued body part.

Alongside my schoolwork, I continued with therapy at the Surrey Treatment Centre, a 24-foot by 60-foot prefabricated building constructed by the Van Zor Grotto, a benevolent organization similar to the Shriners, where I had gone to Kindergarten and therapy the previous year.

The need for services eventually outgrew this tiny facility, and the Variety Club became involved in raising funds for a larger, better-equipped facility. Because I was such a cheerful and cooperative child, the Lower Fraser Valley Cerebral Palsy Association, which operated the Treatment Centre, approached my parents about me being the "star" of that year's Variety Club Telethon.

My parents did not take the decision lightly; in fact, it was quite a dilemma. They appreciated that the telethon raised much needed money for special facilities and equipment for kids with disabilities that the government wouldn't pay for, but they also did not want me to be exploited or used to play on the public's pity. Eventually, they decided the balance weighed in favour of the opportunity to help other kids.

I was very excited because that was the first year Bob MacGrath from Sesame Street was involved with our telethon. I was going to be on TV with Bob MacGrath! How could a six-year-old girl want anything more? Mom miraculously scraped together a few extra dollars to buy me a special blue dress for the occasion.

The telethon was from 7pm Saturday to 6pm Sunday. I was there to open the show, appropriately named the *Show of Hearts* since it is always held near Valentine's Day. I made a couple of appearances later that evening and a few the following day.

Since some celebrities didn't return to their hotels to sleep, a van in which they could rest was parked backstage. I was repeatedly asked if I wanted to go to the van to lie down, but there was no way this six-year-old was going to nap with so much going on! I do remember snuggling up to jazz musician Big Miller's big tummy at one point, though not because I was sleepy! Blake Edmonds jumped around on the phone tables, encouraging viewers to ring those phones. Donors with bagfuls of pennies were received as if they had donated thousands of dollars. There was so much energy and adrenaline pumping. Who could sleep?

By the end of the weekend, if indeed it took that long, I was in love with Bob MacGrath! In fact, I decided I would marry him when I got older! He even signed my red hockey helmet, which I wore while walking. In the eyes of this little redhead, the relationship was getting serious! Since this was long before VCRs were common devices in homes, Mrs. Rutherford took a picture of me on TV to capture the moment. Unfortunately, she ended up with a nice photo of her television set!

Beginning some time around the telethon and continuing for a few years while funding was raised to build the treatment centre, the school principal frequently brought around *looky-loos* to see the Special Ed classes. They were typically people interested in making large donations and educators interested in learning more about kids with special needs. I really felt like we were monkeys in the zoo. They were there only briefly, not long enough to get to know us or really understand us. And they would talk about us as if we weren't there or didn't understand what they were saying about us. After the umpteenth time, I was tempted to fake a seizure or something so that they had something to watch.

With all of us students working at different levels and different curricula, Mrs. Rutherford wrote our daily assignments on small cards that she taped to our desks each morning. That way we would know what to do next if she were busy working with another student. Because Mom was now a teacher down the hall, I was always at school fairly early. Rather than doing nothing as I sat at my desk alone in my classroom, I would start on my day's work. I was finished my morning's work by recess time, so Mrs. Rutherford was soon scrambling to find additional work to keep me busy.

In Grade 4, I had a new teacher, Mrs. Peart, at a *new* school because several of the Special Ed classes were moved over to the main school. Eventually, the annex was torn down, and the lot became a car dealership that stands only blocks from where I'm writing this now.

Being at the main school, our class now had access to the school library. We trekked down the hall to the library once each week to learn about the Dewey Decimal System and to check out a book. After a few weeks, the librarian strongly encouraged me to check out the very limited section of books on tape, assuming that using the newest technology at the time might be easier for me than holding books and turning pages. Honestly, I felt as though she was more concerned that I might crumple the corners as my cp hands turned the pages.

Being a teacher, Mom knew that listening to stories was not the same as reading books. Limiting her bright child to tapes to avoid crumpled corners was not acceptable. Mom, who firmly believes that one catches more flies with honey than with vinegar, politely mentioned to the librarian that I had owned books since I was young and was very careful with them. As a young child, Mom gave me old Sears catalogs to look at so that I learned how to turn the pages without worrying if a page got accidentally torn.

After that one incident, I *read* the entire *Little House on the Prairies* series. I so wanted to be Laura Ingalls, living in a little log house and experiencing her adventures. From there I read books like *Ice Castles* about a talented figure skater who became blind but continued competing by hiding her disability, *The Other Side of the Mountain* about an Olympic-bound skier who broke her neck during a qualifying competition, and *Joni* (pronounced Johnny), who also became a quadriplegic resulting from a diving accident.

Back in Grade 2 or 3, Mrs. Rutherford gave me *Wren,* a children's book about a young girl with cerebral palsy, loosely based on an actual person. It also had illustrations of Wren standing in her long legged braces and crutches. Unlike other children's books, which I enjoyed but didn't identify with because I couldn't see myself in the illustrations, I could relate to the pictures in that small book.

Back then, I didn't know any successful people with disabilities who were much older than me, and I don't recall any people with disabilities in the public eye. These books, particularly the autobiographies, provided me with much needed role models. They showed me what was possible, despite having a disability. It was one thing to have my parents, teachers and therapists tell me to work hard so that I could accomplish anything I wanted. It was another thing to read about adults in wheelchairs who became teachers or got married. I began to realize what was truly possible. Those books planted the seed, when I was about ten, that I would one day write my own story to help others to see what was possible when living with cerebral palsy.

A few years later, in the early 1980s, Geri Jewell made a few guest appearances on the TV series *The Facts of Life*. Geri has cerebral palsy, albeit milder than mine in that she can walk and her speech is fairly clear. She was the first actress with a disability to receive a recurring role on a television show. I thought it was amazing that someone with cp could be an actor on TV, and watching her really opened my mind to possibilities.

Beginning in Grade 4, I was integrated into a regular class in the afternoons – long before *integration* and *mainstreaming* were buzzwords – for Social Studies, Science and Music, the non-core subjects. I soon made friends in that class and looked forward to going to that classroom after lunch.

Around this time, I became friends with David in the regular class. He was new to Canada and had yet to make many friends. We soon became inseparable. He came to my class before school, wheeled me to the regular class after lunch, and then back to my class at the end of the day.

Somehow we joined the choir that practiced during lunch. Considering my speech, it is a funny memory, but it was something David and I could do together during lunch hour. I enjoyed it, although I simply mouthed the words most of the time. The choir performed at the nearby old folks' home and shopping mall, and I vaguely remember a performance on the local cable channel. I didn't enjoy performing because when I am nervous, I tense up, causing my spasticity to increase and making it extremely difficult to hold my head still, which further increases my embarrassment. It's not a pretty sight, but there's nothing I can do about it. One of those times when having cp really sucks. Regardless, when I am home alone, I still enjoy playing Christmas music and passionately singing the traditional carols because it reminds me of good times shared with a special friend.

Grade 5 was also the year of the anticipated sex education film in the regular class. However, on the day of the said film, I was not allowed to go to the regular classroom in the afternoon. I had not returned the required permission slip to see the film because I had not been given a permission slip in the first place. I don't know if it was an oversight, if slips had been handed out in the morning, if I had been sick that day, or if the teachers felt I was not ready for such information and intentionally did not give me a permission slip. Either way, I did not see the film. I thought it was strange since Mom taught down the hall and could have signed the slip *that* day, had she been asked.

The incident was glossed over as no big deal and quickly forgotten; however, I did not forget. Not seeing the film was not as troubling as not receiving permission, for whatever reason, to see the film. Looking back on it, it sent me the message that sex and sexuality were not for me and that I didn't have permission to be involved or to acknowledge that part of myself. This message stuck with me and made me more susceptible to confirmations of that message, even unintentional ones, from family, friends, the media, and society in general. It makes me think of the tongue-in-cheek slogan from the disabled community, "No sex please, we're disabled."

I also wondered what message it sent to my able-bodied classmates and friends. I was allowed to join them for Science and Social Studies, but not for sex ed? Were they not to think of their friends and peers with disabilities as sexual beings? It is strange how an apparently non-significant incident can reverberate through a lifetime.

I was late starting Grade 6 due to my surgery and extended hospitalization. I was so happy to be back in school, despite being in casts. My teacher, who was now Mrs. Rutherford again, had sent home a few textbooks with Mom, including the Grade 6 math text rather than the Grade 5 text, which confused me. I thought Mrs. Rutherford had forgotten that I was a year behind in math because one year I had physiotherapy scheduled after recess a few times a week and missed math class. Mrs. Rutherford had remembered, but she felt that I was capable of handling the Grade 6 materials. It felt good to skip one grade and to be at the level where I should be.

Since I still had to keep my feet up for most of the day, I stayed in my wheelchair at school and did all my work on my wheelchair tray. Mrs. Rutherford lifted my typewriter on and off my tray, as needed. When it was time to learn long division, the typewriter was too cumbersome initially. So, I was given a large sheet of newsprint and worked out the solution in pencil, with an eraser nearby. It took effort to keep the numbers lined up in the correct column and to print legibly enough to work out the solution. I managed to solve only a couple of questions on each large sheet of paper. Gradually, I learned to solve the problem and was allowed to do every other question to save some time and energy.

Once I understood the process, I switched back to using the typewriter for math. Doing long division on an electric typewriter, manually scrolling the page up and down and ensuring the numbers lined up correctly, was a challenge! I'm not sure which was faster – using the pencil or the typewriter! Once the teacher was convinced that I knew what I was doing, she allowed me to use a calculator for some exercises. Mom found me a large calculator with large buttons and a handle so that I could hold it still with my fisted right hand. As I worked through the textbook, checking work with the answers in the back, and then rechecking my work, I discovered many errors in the answer key, confirmed by the teacher. I skipped an entire grade of math and was still able to correct the answer key!

Grade 7 was a bit of a leap and somewhat risky, as I was fully integrated into the regular class for the entire day. Initially, I was nervous and somewhat scared even though I had been with these kids in the afternoons since Grade 4. It meant considerably more time doing homework in order to keep up, but I did manage.

The other kids were very helpful to the four of us in wheelchairs. One lunch hour, the fire alarm went off and, without the bathroom aide or teacher in the room, good-looking James put me in my wheelchair and took me outside. James didn't think twice about it but simply acted responsibly.

An educational chance of a lifetime arose early in the school year. The King Tut exhibition made its way to Seattle. Since we were going to study Egypt at some point that year, the teacher decided to cover that unit first and to go on a field trip to see the timely exhibition. The entire class, plus the bathroom aide and some parents, took the 3-hour Amtrak train ride down to Seattle to experience ancient Egypt. I found it completely fascinating to see artifacts from ancient times from a far, far away land. Totally awesome! It was an extremely long day, but well worth it.

That was also the first time I experienced a food court in a shopping mall. There was such a choice of food in one place that it was difficult to choose what I wanted for lunch. I think I chose spaghetti. I have since learned to choose the least messy meal when dining out, even if something else sounds more tempting.

Within a couple of months, the school needed a full-time vice-principal; much to our disappointment, we lost our great teacher. Another one was hired to fill his position. We quickly discovered that our new teacher had some *unconventional* teaching methods, which caused a few waves. His first day he came in and ripped down all of the spelling tests from the wall. I don't know if he felt we were too old to have work up on the wall or if he wanted the space for something else. Either way, I felt it was hurtful and disrespectful. Things didn't improve from there. Being typical Grade 7 kids, we soon had a few choice nicknames for him. As far as I know, his teaching contract was not renewed at the end of the year.

But, he did have us do one exercise regularly to get us writing. He would pick a word, like *cars*, and we had five minutes to write as much as we could about cars. I think the purpose was to get us over the fear of putting words down on paper and to get thoughts flowing. On a couple of occasions, as a replacement assignment if there was something I couldn't do, he had me pick one moment or incident and write as much as I could about it by describing all of my five senses. The idea was to expand that one moment in time as much as possible and to include as many details as I could remember.

I still use those techniques if I'm stuck while writing. I start writing to get the ideas flowing and to get *something* down on paper. From there, I can go back to pick out the portions worth keeping, and then I can proceed. Despite him not being my favourite teacher, I do remember him for encouraging my writing, and I do owe him some gratitude. Perhaps he saw potential and knew that writing would have to play an important part in my life.

On the last day of Grade 7, Mom wheeled me out to the van like she did every other day. There were a few tears as we passed Mrs. Peart in her classroom. She gave me a gift that I still have to this day – a butterfly necklace, symbolizing freedom in a new life. And then Mom and I left, not to return, as it was the last day for the both of us. Mom had resigned her teaching position so that she would be available to assist me in high school; a risky move financially and professionally but one that she felt was necessary to give me the best chance of success.

We went through those doors, neither one of us certain of what the next chapter would bring but knowing we would get through it, one way or another.

Guiding Lights

My childhood was not all traumatic hospital stays; in fact, I remember it being fairly *normal*. In Grade 3, my best friend Sandy joined Brownies, so, naturally, I also *had* to join. I kept bugging Mom until she made the necessary phone calls. Living in a different city from Sandy, Mom called the Commissioner in our home district to check out the possibility of a girl with physical disabilities joining Brownies. The Commissioner said they had never had a Brownie in a wheelchair in the district, possibly the region; but after a long conversation with Mom, she was willing to give it a shot and let me join.

I soon enrolled in the Brownie Pack closest to our home. This was a welcomed change after having to cross school district boundaries to attend a school that was equipped to educate me. Yet, a group of volunteers with no Special Ed experience was willing to give me an opportunity to learn, grow and have fun with girls in my own home community. This was the first time, yet definitely not the only time, that I found people outside the "helping" professions more helpful, which amazes me. These people are actually angels here on earth.

One year before I was integrated half-time into a regular class at school, I participated in regular Brownie meetings held in a local elementary school gym, only blocks from home. I was the only one with a disability in the pack, but no one seemed to notice. Soon the other girls were fighting over who could push my little, red wheelchair. While the girls viewed this as a special privilege, one girl in particular, Karen, saw it as *her* duty, so the others had few chances. She and I became inseparable, and we did everything together in Brownies. She saw beyond my cp for whom I truly was, and our friendship was one that lasted through our Guiding years and beyond. Our lives have taken us on different paths, but they have crossed again at various junctures. I hope this special friendship will still be there when we are old and grey, and we can look back and remember our times together.

Mom worked closely with Brown Owl and the other Guiders to adapt the program requirements, where necessary, to ensure any changes were fair and required the same effort from me. For example, one requirement was to jump rope for a minimum of ten jumps. Obviously, jumping rope was not possible for me. Mom suggested that I be required to wheel my manual wheelchair, something I seldom did independently as it required much effort, a specified distance. Brown Owl agreed that it was a fair substitute.

When it came to sewing on a button, Mom put a small embroidery hoop on an old sock and found a few large buttons from her mom's button jar. She handed me a darning needle and, with much effort and a few jabs into my thigh, I sewed on two buttons, by myself, making a sock puppet.

To light a candle, I used a long fireplace match and a piece of sandpaper temporarily taped to my wheelchair tray. Mom steadied my arm as a fire safety precaution since a jerky arm with a lit match could have been disastrous. I don't light candles often, but I do think of alternate ways of doing things, which was the key to my experiences. I learned to think outside of the box and to come up with solutions when others may have said it was not possible and would not have enabled me to try.

Another Brownie requirement for completing the program was to learn finger spelling, the alphabet used by people who are hearing impaired or deaf. This was something we learned as a pack, and we each carried the alphabet card in our uniform pockets. I had just enough hand function to manage forming each letter reasonably well, which was fantastic because it suddenly gave me a simple way of communicating a few words with everyone in the pack without any cumbersome communication devices. To this day, when I am orally spelling a word that someone is having difficulty understanding, I often find myself finger spelling the word as well.

When I was allowed to use a calculator in school, my parents bought an alphanumeric calculator for me. They thought I could use it for communication when people didn't know finger spelling even if it was limited to only eight letters at a time. Unlike other communication devices at that time, it was small enough to slip into my pocket, so I took that to Brownies as well. My friends liked to decipher the letters as some were rather cryptic in the confined calculator space.

In the spring, the pack headed off to Brownie camp at the Odd Fellows Lodge in oceanside White Rock, enjoying a weekend of hiking, exploring the beach, making crafts, and singing camp songs. And, of course, I went too. That was never a question. Mom volunteered as a camp cook so that she would be available when I needed assistance. I remember we Brownies had the responsibility of giving the two cooks camp names with the only stipulation being that the names must be food. We gleefully came up with *Nuts* and *Crackers*, and this redhead had her hand in the decision! Mom was known as *Nuts* during the entire weekend.

I had my fair share of KP duty, standing at the sink and washing tons of dishes with my friend Karen. We also had our turn at setting the tables. Years later, I visited Karen's house for a large family gathering, and her mom asked the two of us to set the long table. Obviously, she remembered me capably setting the tables at camp, so she expected me to do my part to assist with the family dinner. I did it gladly while humming a line from a camp song, "There is a duty to be done, and I say I." It felt good to be included and to be expected to do my part.

At camp Mom learned an important lesson: to sit on her hands as I tried to do something by myself, even if it took me longer to accomplish. Like most moms, time was in great demand. She worked full-time, raised four kids and kept the household running, and she didn't always have the luxury of time to allow me to do something myself that she could do more quickly. However, she knew it was critical to allow me to do what I could myself, even if it took longer, in order to develop independence.

The Guiders taught Mom to sit on her hands whenever possible rather than rushing in to do things for me, but reality meant some compromises. On school day mornings, when timing was down to the minute, she dressed me. But, on weekends when we didn't have to be anywhere early, I dressed myself, even though it could take half an hour or more. Who invented socks anyway? They were always a struggle, but I managed to get them on eventually. Because I preferred doing things myself rather than having others do them for me, I was nicknamed the "I'll-do-it-myself" girl.

Following the morning events of one Thinking Day, which honoured Lord and Lady Baden-Powell as the founders of the Guiding and Scouting movements, my family, still in our various uniforms, attended the final hours of the Variety Club Telethon. In the next day's newspaper there was a photo of me watching the telethon, but my excitement was quickly extinguished when I read the caption, which referred to me as a *he* enjoying the show. The paper referred to me, in my Brownie uniform, as a he.

I was indignant! I thumped on my knees, my method of mobility at home, down the hall to my bedroom, stuck a sheet of paper in my electric typewriter and typed a letter to the newspaper editor, explaining that I couldn't possibly be a boy as I was clearly wearing a Brownie uniform. Dad delivered my letter to the newspaper office the following day. The man apologized to me through Dad, offering a lame excuse about a typesetting error. How can you run a newspaper if you can't get the facts straight and don't check for errors? Even though I never received an adequate response, it taught me to stand up for myself when I felt I had been wronged.

At age eleven, with the Brownie program completed and our *Golden Hands* earned, Karen and I and a few others *flew* up to Guides, an intimidating move because we were now the youngest girls in this seemingly much older group. But we soon adjusted. For instance, I learned that the Colour Party wasn't actually a colouring party. How was I to know it referred to the flag bearers and their guards?

Unfortunately, my time as an actual Girl Guide was short-lived because, in the fall of 1979, Girl Guides of Canada changed the ages for Brownies and Guides and introduced a new program called Pathfinders for my age group. I was disappointed as I had less than a year to earn a few badges and to plan out how I was going to earn the All Round Cord, the then second highest award a girl could earn in Guides, second to the Canada Cord.

I was bothered only until I started with Pathfinders and developed a new plan. I have always felt more content and fulfilled when working towards a goal, even though the work may be hard or frustrating at times. I think the Guiding program was good for that reason because it rewarded girls for working towards and reaching goals. I learned to plan and to organize by using self-discipline to stay focused. Or, perhaps I had those natural abilities, and the Guiding program enabled and encouraged me to use them. Either way, it was important training for later in life.

Keeping up with an increasing homework load with one typing thumb in my high school years unfortunately meant I missed a fair number of Pathfinder meetings. At one point I had to switch Pathfinder Units, and Karen didn't switch with me, so our paths began going separate ways. Childhood friendships change and evolve over time, which is part of growing up. Sometimes they change for the good, and sometimes for the sad. Pathfinders wasn't quite the same as Brownies; however, I did participate as much as my school load permitted, including outings and weekend camping trips.

One memorable outing was the morning of March 9, 1983. Our Guiders had arranged for our Pathfinder Unit to be present when Queen Elizabeth II was welcomed to Vancouver on the steps of City Hall. We arrived hours ahead of time to wait in line, in the cold. My entire family was there, dressed in our various Guiding and Scouting uniforms.

As I was in my wheelchair, I was allowed to sit, alongside the senior citizens, directly behind the rope that lined the route the Queen would take on her walkabout while the rest of the Pathfinders stood behind me and the others in wheelchairs. Mom had picked up a bouquet at Safeway, *just in case*. With my lack of voluntary hand control, especially at the most inopportune times, I envisioned having a tug-of-war with the Queen over the bouquet of flowers. Subsequently, the Pathfinder behind me was primed, if necessary, to reach over to steady my arm.

I also envisioned my feet flying off my footrests in a moment of excitement and kicking Her Majesty in the shins. I could see myself being tackled by secret servicemen. To avoid that scene, I decided to tuck my feet behind the footrests to hold my feet still. In the worst-case scenario, I would end up with small bruises on *my* shins from bashing them on the metal footrests, but I figured it was a small price to pay to be that close to the Queen.

Finally, the time came for her to begin her walkabout. She came walking down the red carpet towards me. She saw me holding the flowers, and she stopped and asked, "Are those for me?" Trembling, I replied, "Yes." My arm moved gracefully for someone with cp, and my hand opened with ease. She took the bouquet and said, "Thank you," before continuing down the line. I had given flowers to the Queen! I was so excited!

Prince Philip also stopped to say something to us Pathfinders. As I was still in awe of having given flowers to the Queen without any mishaps, I didn't hear what he said to us. The next day the Vancouver newspaper had a beautiful colour photo on the front page of the Queen with an armful of bouquets, including mine, still wrapped in

Safeway cellophane. Once the Royal couple and their entourage drove away, freeing us to move, the Pathfinders handed out the potted flowers that had lined the City Hall steps to the seniors in wheelchairs; a fitting memento of the special occasion.

The six Watsons then piled into our van and headed to BC Place Stadium, which was still under construction and scheduled to open officially in three months. At that time, it was North America's largest air-supported dome stadium, and seeing the new air-pressurized stadium was an amazing experience. I remember Neal's Scout beret blowing off as we left because of the difference in air pressure between the inside and outside, which was necessary to keep up the unsupported fiberglass woven fabric dome.

Mom had scored special tickets from the radio station to be at BC Place when the Queen invited the world to Expo '86. She rarely pulled us out of school, particularly when I was in high school, except for medical appointments, but she felt this was a special exception, a chance of a lifetime. She felt it was a unique educational experience, so she ran for the phone when she heard the announcement on the radio.

After another seemingly long wait, the Royal couple arrived in an open car and drove around the perimeter of the field. Following speeches from various dignitaries, Her Majesty officially invited the world to Vancouver for Expo '86. On a large world map overhead, we watched countries light up as dignitaries placed phone calls relaying the Queen's invitation.

After making the Brownie and Guide promises for years "to do my duty to … the Queen," it was quite an experience to see her in person and to hand her a bouquet of flowers. The experience piqued my already keen interest in the Royal family, as I read whatever books I could and watched Royal events on television.

I slowly worked on the Pathfinder program, in between homework assignments, and I eventually completed the requirements for all five emblems: Home, Community, World, Outdoors and Camping. My final major challenge was to plan and organize a camping weekend for a small group of Pathfinders. I did everything from planning menus and quarter mastering to designing compass games and assigning camp chores. I don't know if it was my obsessive attention to detail or my controlling nature, but I had everything planned in detail on paper. Although it was a fair bit of work, I enjoyed the planning process. In the end, I realized the key was to keep the four of us dry, fed and happy, even if it meant not everything was executed as planned. We had a good time, with no significant mishaps.

With the camp challenge successfully under my belt, I had completed the requirements for the distinguished Canada Cord and was presented it at the Mother-Daughter Banquet, with my whole family in attendance. That was a proud and exciting moment, showing once again that I could accomplish anything I put my mind to and persevered. Having completed that chapter in Guiding, I then moved up to the next program, Cadets, a junior leadership-training program.

That July, Kevin went with his Scout troop to the World Jamboree (WJ '83) in Kananaskis, outside of Banff, Alberta. The rest of our family camped not far from the jamboree site so that we could visit a few times during the ten-day event. On our first visit, as we were walking along the main road of the tent city towards Kevin's campsite, which was at the opposite end of the main gate about a mile away, it started pouring rain.

Mom was pushing me in my manual wheelchair, and she headed for the nearest shelter, which, coincidentally, was the Finnish contingent's dining shelter. I had been writing to a Finnish penpal, Pãivi, since the summer of 1979. She was also in the Guiding movement, though she wasn't there at the jamboree. Meeting some Finns in person and hearing their accents seemed to bring Pãivi's letters alive on another dimension.

We spoke to the leaders as we dried off and waited for the rain to stop. We spoke about my Guiding experiences and how I had recently earned my Canada Cord. The leaders told us more about Finland and about their Scouting program, which was co-ed like many programs are throughout the world. The head leader, who I think was the National Commissioner, personally invited me to their international camp Miilu '85. Even though it was still two years away, I was excited. In addition to new experiences, it meant that I might finally meet Pãivi. I now had to work to make this new dream a reality.

That evening we stayed for the Opening Ceremony. Moments before they began, the skies opened up and the heavens fell, soaking everyone. Several Scout troops found their tents in instant rivers and scrambled to grab their belongings before they floated away. A beautiful rainbow appeared, centered perfectly above the outside stage. The Irish Rovers started playing and troubles were forgotten. The Scouts from Britain and Northern Ireland crossed their flags in friendship – if only the youth ruled the world. The Dutch went by doing the Congo line, stopping briefly to pour the water from their wooden shoes. Wasn't that a party!

Walking along the main camp road another day, an American Scout leader noticed that I didn't yet have a miniature, carved wooden boot from the Ozarks on my camp hat covered in crests and pins, so he pinned one on. The boot swung on its short, leather lace, gently bonking me on the head every time my chair hit a rock, which, on a gravel road, was constantly. We walked so much that week that my solid rubber tires were worn down; bits of rubber were flaking off of them. Solid rubber tires, by the way, have no shock absorbency and can be rather tiresome on the butt. The thin piece of foam on a piece of plywood simply dulled the teeth-rattling bumps. But I didn't care. I enjoyed meeting people from around the world and learning how they lived.

That September, as a Cadet, I began volunteering as a junior leader with a Brownie Pack. Again, homework took precedence and attendance at meetings was sporadic. The actual Cadet program was done by correspondence, thus I was able to gradually complete those assignments during breaks in my homework. Having never met my Cadet advisor face-to-face, I once again needed self-discipline to stay motivated and focused to complete the program. It also meant that I didn't have contact with other Cadets, so it was somewhat isolating not sharing the experiences with other girls my own age.

In a somewhat surprise presentation at the end of the school year, I was honoured with the Girl Guide of Canada's Badge of Fortitude. In her congratulatory letter, the Chief Commissioner wrote that my determination to do my best, considering my limitations, was indeed living the then eighth Guide Law, "A Guide smiles and sings even under difficulty."

Most days I didn't see my cp as a limitation, and I surely didn't see myself as courageous or inspirational, as others claimed. But it was nice to be recognized for working hard, even though I didn't view what I had done as extraordinary. I simply lived my life. I wasn't using my cp as an excuse for not working hard, doing my best, and living my life to its fullest.

That evening our Member of Parliament, Benno Friessen, was unable to attend; he sent his wife in his place and had her read William Wordsworth's *Nuns Fret Not*. That sonnet struck a chord with me, and I have read it occasionally through the years. Even though others see my disability as restrictive and limiting, I am like the nuns, hermits and poets in his poem. I am quite content, for the most part, with my life. Of course, I always want to better myself as a person and to accomplish more, but I don't consider myself confined by my cerebral palsy.

At the same time, I was also presented with the Bertha Mabel Somerville Citizenship Prize, a cash award. I opened my first savings account, which became my seed money for the international camp in Finland in a year's time. My dream of meeting my penpal was beginning to become reality. I then began selling Regal Greetings and did some work for my Dad over the summer. Between the money I earned and the money from various levels of Girl Guides of Canada, I raised enough for my trip.

Somehow my family managed to pull enough money together for Mom to accompany me, although it was a financially bleak time for us. For a while, we had a 4-foot by 10-foot drying rack hanging on pulleys from our family room ceiling because there was no money to fix the dryer. My parents figured that if I had worked hard to do my part, then they weren't going to let me miss the opportunity.

This time I wasn't merely a visitor, an observer, but a full-fledged camp participant who had earned her way there, signified by the camp scarf. Mom and I went with the

Canadian contingent of Girl Guides. Our small group camped with a Finnish Guide and Scout troop, giving us the opportunity to learn more about the Finnish culture, while they learned more about Canada from us. Camping with blonde-haired, blue-eyed guys everywhere, albeit in separate tents, was heavenly!

The washhouse, nicknamed the Plastic Palace within our group, was quite an experience. The "toilets" were two 2 x 4 boards across large plastic garbage cans partly filled with sawdust that were emptied regularly. For someone with tenuous balance (and an overactive gag reflex), teetering my skinny butt between these two boards took concentration; otherwise, the consequences would have been unspeakable.

The cold running water was fine for brushing teeth and washing faces, but was a little more than *refreshing* for showering. Thankfully, the organizers had arranged for the International leaders and the few campers in wheelchairs to use the shower and sauna facilities at the small airport nearby. Sometimes having a disability has its advantages!

A camp volunteer drove Mom and I and another fellow in a wheelchair to the airport every few days. The women's shower was one large room with showerheads along the perimeter walls. There were no partitions or curtains, so women of all shapes and sizes were walking around naked and uninhibited. Being from uptight North America, this was all new to me. With no shower bench, there was no place for me to sit to shower except for the floor. As I sat there doing my thing with naked women all around, I felt like I was in an x-rated movie! I used Mom's honey-glycerin soap for the first time and ended up with an intensely itchy rash in places that aren't polite to scratch. It was then I learned one should not try new soap while camping in a foreign country, as remedies for allergic reactions may not be readily available.

The evening of the Opening Ceremony was chilly; after all, we were only a few hundred miles from the Arctic Circle. Thankfully, Mom brought a Teflon rescue suit, similar to the rescue blankets I was wrapped in when we went snowshoeing as a family, in case I became cold while we were camping. Wearing this silver tinfoil suit and Finnish mitts we bought during our few days in Helsinki, I felt like an alien from outer space. Despite looking extremely odd, I managed to keep fairly warm that evening as thousands of us came together on a hillside to experience the ceremony the Finnish way.

After corresponding for four years, on Visitors' Day I finally met my penpal Pãivi and her family. I was so excited! I had purchased two small teddy bears with Canada t-shirts to give to Pãivi and her little brother Timo on this occasion. After the jamboree, Mom and I had an extended homestay with her family in Oulu. They were gracious hosts, showing us many sights around the area and introducing us to their family and friends. Apparently, it is Finnish tradition to serve seven goodies when entertaining, and it's impolite not to eat one of each. I did my utmost best not to be rude! They even took us on an overnight trip to Santa's Village at the Arctic Circle and over to a small border town in Sweden. They forgot that we were Canadians and that we should have driven through the Customs lane. Ooops! I simply omitted that side-trip from my written report to Girl Guide Headquarters!

There were a few tears as Mom and I boarded the train back to Helsinki to rejoin the Canadian contingent before going home. Somewhere along the way, the train stopped, seemingly out in nowhere. Since Mom and I didn't speak

Finnish, we weren't sure what was happening. We followed everyone off the train, which was no simple feat with my wheelchair, duffle bag and various bits and pieces. We seemed to be walking towards waiting buses. A young, blonde-haired, blue-eyed Finnish soldier saw we were struggling and helped us, which I didn't mind at all. Through his broken English and our non-existent Finnish, we learned there had been an accident further along the track, and we had to take a bus around the accident and then board another train. So much for a hassle-free train ride enjoying foreign countryside! *Kiitos* to the unnamed Finnish soldier.

Returning to our new home in the Cariboo in the interior of British Columbia, I continued the Cadet program and volunteering with a Brownie Pack, of which Mom was the Brown Owl. The two of us ran the group for about one year. For my final Cadet challenge, I planned a Brownie Revel "Brownies in Action '86: Guiding Sisters Working Together", a fun day for the district. Again it was no simple task, but I planned everything down to the smallest detail and then handed my binder over to the District Commissioner for her to put into action.

At the day's closing, I was presented with the Cadet 'C' pin, signifying that I had completed the Cadet program and, essentially, the Guiding program. The next step would have been to participate more at the adult level, but circumstances didn't facilitate that at that point in my life. I chose to end my Guiding involvement after such a full career.

Horsing Around

When I was in Grade 4, the Treatment Centre arranged for a few classmates and me to take some horseback riding lessons with the Pacific Riding for the Disabled Association (PRDA). The physios felt it would be a good form of therapy as well as a recreational activity for us. This was the beginning of something wonderful!

A mini-school bus picked us up after school and took us to the riding stables. Each of us was assigned to a horse. Mine was Tater, a 16 hands high Palomino with a golden blonde mane and tail. Since a hand is four inches, he was no small pony! My legs reached only part way down his sides. Three volunteers were assigned to each rider – one to lead the horse and two side-handlers to support the rider as needed. For safety we each wore a wide, leather waist belt for the side-handlers to use to support us or to grab if something should go wrong. In addition, for trotting and posting we held onto the neck strap, a thin strap loosely around the horse's neck. This saved us from inadvertently pulling on the horse's mouth. It also gave us a bit more stability. And, of course, we wore English riding helmets.

In the beginning, as Mom so poignantly described it, I looked like a rag doll atop the horse. My head would flop, my trunk control was tenuous, and my hands could barely hang on to the reins. Even so, I had a great big smile on my face. This was the beginning of my love affair with horses!

After each lesson, we thanked the horses by feeding them carrots. A volunteer held our hands flat so that no curled fingers got in the way of those big teeth. We then drank hot chocolate and ate cookies before heading home. At home I practiced grasping the reins with a dog leash wrapped around my bedpost. Soon I was able to hold them correctly, with the slight modification of knots tied in the reins to keep them from slipping through my small hands when Tater pulled his big head.

    Our riding instructor was an actual English riding instructor, Aunty Jo, who donated her time to the program. She was strict, expecting us to work hard and to do our best, yet she was fun. She joked about putting an ice cream cone between Tater's ears, and every time I wasn't looking straight forward she would take a lick of ice cream.

    Shortly, I had the correct posture of a rider – head up, shoulders back, back straight and heels down. The side-handlers no longer had to support me while we were walking. Trotting, however, was a different matter. My head bounced around so much that I didn't really like trotting. The physio, who occasionally watched the lessons, suggested trying a soft neck brace to support my neck; one suggestion that actually worked.

    One time the National Adjudicator came to assess the program for insurance purposes. At one point during the lesson, we were going over very low jumps. During my turn, my helmet flew off, hitting Tater on the rump and causing him to buck. The side-handlers grabbed my waist belt and pulled me off. The horsehandler walked Tater around a bit, calming him down. Then Aunty Jo had me get back on before fear set in. The class carried on.

    Aunty Jo was so upset that the incident had to occur during the adjudicator's visit. Mom tried reassuring her that it was probably a good thing because it demonstrated to the adjudicator that she and the volunteers were able to handle a potentially dangerous situation calmly. The adjudicator passed the program, much to Aunty Jo's relief. The only recommendation was that full chin guards and straps be put on the helmets; a recommendation implemented by the next week's lesson.

The last lesson of the session was a *horse show*. We had competitions and were awarded fancy horse ribbons, which I promptly hung along the window valance in my bedroom.

I continued riding through the years, and I had an ever-growing collection of horse posters, books and ornaments in my room. Cloverdale Feed & Tack became my favourite store.

At some point, riding lessons switched from after school to Saturday mornings. By then, we had moved a little closer to the barn. Moving to a one-level rancher was cheaper than installing an elevator for me. Mom would drive me down, and we would spend the morning at the barn. After the lessons, Aunty Jo often came by for a lunch of tomato soup and ham croissants.

During this time, we also had an arrangement with the horse's owner that allowed me to ride whenever I wished. Mom and I spent many evenings at the barn, grooming, tacking and riding. The all-black barn kitty, which I named Panther, would sit on my lap as soon as I was out of the car into my wheelchair. He took every opportunity to jump up for a cuddle and purr, and I so wanted to take him home with me. Of course, on Christmas mornings I had to go down to give carrots to the horse. Those were happy times.

Through the years, we were actively involved in the PRDA. My brothers were recruited to help bag and sell manure for fundraisers. We lost my baby brother Ian in one pile, and Mom swears he had a significant growth spurt shortly afterwards.

At some point in Grade 8, the National Film Board of Canada filmed a short documentary of the PRDA to use for purposes of training and promotion. Someone suggested me as the main storyline for the documentary. Of course, I didn't object! I found the behind-the-scenes process fascinating, such as the day the crew was filming at our house and had to turn off our refrigerator so that its motor couldn't be heard on the sound recording. That experience planted my still-present itch to work behind the scenes on a *real* movie one day.

As the film was to depict my first riding lesson, I had to do a bit of acting since I had been riding for several years by then. But I didn't mind because it allowed me more time riding Devil Boy. One filming session was virtually an entire day of me riding alone, without the class. Could a young girl want anything more than a whole day of riding solo, in front of the camera? Shooting was done at the posh Southlands Riding Club in Vancouver, which was more picturesque and involved riding in the outdoor arena, which I loved, as well as the green meadow, which was a new experience for me.

The film's last scene depicts the three handlers letting go and setting me free to ride independently, something I had been doing for awhile. But the new challenge for me was keeping Devil Boy from pulling his big head down to munch on the tempting green grass and potentially pulling me off in the process, which would not have been a cool moment to catch on tape!

We even filmed a day at high school. I was remarkably *popular* that day. However, it was decided that those shots did not fit with the film's story, and thus, were omitted from the final cut. We teased my aide Barb that her film debut ended up on the cutting room floor, but it was all good fun.

Because I was Aunty Jo's student and because the film was shot at Southlands with their PRDA group, there was tension between the groups, resulting in some hurt feelings. I felt a bit guilty, like I had caused the tension by agreeing to be involved with the documentary. But a kid can't be responsible for the behaviour of adults.

Shortly after the film was completed, Aunty Jo retired to the interior of British Columbia. Although I never heard from her again, I never forgot her. Today, when driving along the sidewalk in my scooter, I often think, "back straight, shoulders back, head up and eyes straight ahead." I imagine looking between the horse's ears; otherwise, Aunty Jo will take a lick of the ice cream cone.

She gave me a new sense of freedom and independence, as well as a new perspective of the world, in a way that no one else could. Being atop a horse, I could separate myself from my wheelchair, which, although it enables me mobility, it symbolizes my disability. People instantly know I have a disability when seeing me in my wheelchair, and they approach (or avoid) me based on the stereotypes, assumptions and misconceptions they have about people with disabilities. On the horse, at first glance they do not see my cp in all its jerky, gross, misunderstood ways. For that brief moment, until they take a closer look or interact with me, my disability does not exist. They simply see me. That is the sense of freedom I feel atop of the horse.

I was riding independently – with no horsehandler and no side-handlers – long before I had my first electric scooter. Horseback riding was a recreational activity that I *could do*, not something else I had to sit on the sidelines and watch. And, when friends were talking about horses, particularly in high school, I could join in the conversation.

Thank you, Aunty Jo. Wherever you are, I will always remember you and all that you taught me.

Our local PRDA group participated in a few parades to promote awareness of riding for people with disabilities. I took part in these events, eagerly accepting any opportunity to ride. One that I vividly recall was the Steveston Salmon Festival Parade on July 1, 1982, in which the Black Powder group followed a few entries behind us. Every time they fired off a blank, our horses would spook a little. Keeping Devil Boy under control along the lengthy parade route, while trying to smile the entire way, took some extra effort. Being unusually tired when we got home, I had a nap, which was rare for me. I awoke to discover I had entered womanhood. Oh, Happy Canada Day!

July of 1983 was another big moment in my riding career. The BC Summer Games decided to include equestrian events for people with disabilities as a demonstration sport. I decided to ride in the Kur class, which was the freestyle class.

Together with my coach Regan and my side-handler Cheryl, we came up with a program to ride. I chose John Denver's "Sweet Surrender" as my music, not the traditional music for an English Kur, but the song spoke to me. Susan generously allowed me to ride Devil Boy for this venture, too. I wanted to be sure I knew the program by heart; in fact, I practiced it while in my electric scooter whenever I had a large enough empty space.

The Games finally arrived. The first evening was the Opening Ceremony and the Parade of Athletes. I had fun lining up with all the other athletes from across the province, parading around the track, and then sitting on the field as comrades during the rest of the Ceremony.

Dad remembers that moment well. Standing there with his three *healthy* sons, he was watching his *disabled* daughter parade with the other athletes, thinking something was wrong with this picture. Dad, we were simply a family supporting one another's interests. What is wrong with that? Isn't that what being a family is all about? A couple weeks previously we were camping in Kananaskis, outside of Banff, Alberta, so that we could visit the World Jamboree, which Kevin was attending with his Scout troop.

Back at our campsite, I met a mountain climber who had climbed Mount Everest. Although he didn't reach *the* summit, he did reach *his* summit. When I told him I was going to be in my first competition in the upcoming BC Summer Games, he gave me one of his climbing clips so that I could reach *my* summit. I wore the clip on a blue ribbon under my wool blazer, which my friend Karen's mom found for me at a consignment store.

I was slightly nervous as I entered the ring and bowed to the judges. But soon it was Devil Boy, my music and me. Everything else disappeared. It was a great feeling, one of complete freedom and independence. I was in complete control of the horse, and he was listening to me. I simply did my thing, with Devil Boy as my partner. I rode my five-minute program without a flaw, matching the length of the song, which meant I had paced myself well.

At the end of my program, I halted in the middle of the ring to bow again to the judges. Protocol says you exit the ring by riding to the wall and along the perimeter to the gate. Well, Devil Boy took the opportunity of halting to stand in a perfect show stance, with his hind legs out behind him. No matter how I squeezed my legs, kicked or said "walk on", he would not budge. I suppose he figured since I had five minutes, he deserved a moment to show off, too. Despite what Regan had drilled into me, I finally yanked on the left rein and did an 180° Western-style turn and exited the ring.

Once the two classes were done, the officials were wondering how to get the wheelchairs onto the small podium for the medal presentation; a question that obviously had not occurred to them prior to this moment. Dad suggested that, since we were still on our horses, we simply ride in and stand in front of the appropriate position at the podium. Great idea! We would maintain the same level of independence for the medal presentation as we had during the competition. And the wheelchairs wouldn't distract from the abilities that had been demonstrated on that beautiful afternoon. Perfect!

They told Dad to direct me to the middle position. Isn't the middle position gold? I had won gold! Oh, what a feeling! What a high! I instantly forgot that I was melting in my wool blazer in the hot, mid-afternoon sun. I beamed from ear to ear for the rest of the week!

The following year's Games were held in Burnaby, an urban city next door to Vancouver, which didn't have appropriate facilities for any equestrian events; thus, none were held. I was a bit disappointed that I could not experience the opportunity to compete again with the rest of the young athletes from across the province.

In the subsequent year, the equestrian events for riders with disabilities were added to the BC Summer Games for People with Disabilities. As I had worked hard to work my way out of a Special Ed class into a regular class full-time and then into my neighbourhood high school, I didn't agree with the concept of segregated Summer Games. I felt that if all athletes trained and practiced to the best of their abilities, then they should have the opportunity to compete together, even if it's in separate events. So, I decided not to participate in those Games.

Sometimes I have wondered how far I could have gone as a competitor, but I do not regret my decision. I stood for something I strongly believed in – the same way that I believe the Olympics and Paralympics should be one event, not segregated. I had my one special moment in the ring, *my summit*, and I don't think that feeling could be duplicated. That one moment holds a special place in my memory, and perhaps that is how it should remain.

High School

While in Grade 7, arrangements were made for me to attend our local high school, Seaquam (pronounced see-ACK-kum). Grudgingly, I had testing sessions with the district psychologist to prove to the high school principal and staff that I was capable of handling the regular curriculum. This was not fair; after all, testing was not required of my classmates, yet I had to prove my abilities to adults once again. However, Dr. Kryderman confirmed what my parents, my teachers and I knew all along, so it was no big surprise.

Once the school agreed to register me for the fall, Mom and I met with Miss Brown, who would be my guidance counselor. She showed us around the rather large school. I was impressed by both the lengthy, three-level switchback ramp in the cafeteria, which was the accessible route to the second floor, and the gigantic cookies made by the cafeteria class. What else was important at that age? Surely not course selection and electives!

In June, Mom resigned her teaching position in order to assist me at school with certain activities, such as getting from class to class, taking notes, and going to the bathroom. She accompanied me on the first few days of high school. While it wasn't the *normal* way to start high school, it was a bit of a relief to me since I knew nobody at the new school. Mom and I were more like best friends than mother and daughter. For the most part, we had fun together.

During the second or third week of school, a full-time aide was hired for me. Barb was in her mid-twenties, had her Masters in Special Ed and was hired to assist me in any way needed. Mom was amazed and thrilled! Upon meeting her, I remember Mom asking to pinch her to make sure she was real. After a few days of transition, Barb and I became an inseparable team.

Barb was with me from the time Mom dropped me off in the morning until she picked me up after school. She wheeled me from class to class, up and down that long ramp several times each day. She lifted my typewriter, which I carried with me on my small wheelchair tray, onto the desk in each class. And she took my class notes. She also attempted to calm any fears the teachers had about having a student with cp in their classroom, which was no doubt the most challenging part of her job at times.

I took English, Social Studies, Science and Math. For obvious reasons, I had a waiver for Physical Education and French. Since English combined with *Glenda-ish* was difficult enough, they didn't want to add another language to the mix. In Grade 8, Home Economics or Industrial Arts was also mandatory; they opted to put me with a hot stove rather than power tools. Given the choice, it was probably the safest option for everyone!

Home Ec was fun. There were four of us per cooking unit, and we played the typical teenaged jokes like switching the salt with the sugar so that the next class had a nasty tasting surprise. And, then there was the pizza crust made with one cup of salt rather than one tablespoon. Whoops! We didn't receive a favourable grade for that particular assignment.

Halfway through the year we switched from cooking to sewing. As there was no way I could cut and sew a garment without major hands-on assistance, in which case it wouldn't really be my work, Mom proposed that I do a needlework project. The teacher agreed to the idea. I did a cross-stitch on a "large holed" fabric, using a darning needle. However, I still had to do all the textbook and theory work for the sewing section, one example of how education isn't always useful or practical. I did get an A in the course, which proved you don't always have "to do" in order "to know".

Because I only took five courses out of a possible eight, I had three spare blocks that I used for doing homework since it took me so much longer to type my assignments. I still did hours of homework every night and every weekend in order to keep up with the pace of the courses. While I never turned in a late assignment or asked for an extension, I did make sacrifices, particularly in later grades, as the workload got even heavier. I missed out on doing things with friends that may have been as important to personal development as spending hours on homework. Looking back, I'm not sure if I would do things quite the same way again. Although, with a computer and word prediction software rather than an electric typewriter, I could have done my work more efficiently; thus, saving me from typing a rough draft of a paper and then a good copy. Perhaps I could have done my best on my homework and still have had time to be with friends rather than being in my bedroom most of my high school years.

Occasionally, I escaped my cell. At the end of October came the Halloween Dance – my first high school dance! I was excited! However, because I was still in my manual wheelchair, this posed a minor problem. I needed a pusher, and, in case I needed to go to the bathroom, it had to be a female pusher. Barb was unavailable that night, so, naturally, Mom filled in. I dressed as Santa with a cardboard sleigh, created as a family effort, attached to my chair. Mom was dressed as a toy sack behind me, and she wore a red, yarn wig to look like a Ragedy Ann doll within the sack. I took my Mom, dressed as an old bag, to my first high school dance! Not the *norm*, but everyone was cool with it.

During the fall, I discovered high school basketball, particularly the senior boys' team. I went to several evening and weekend games at the school, sometimes coercing my brother Kevin to go with me. One day before the lunch bell rang, the principal announced that the senior boys had an afternoon game in Abbotsford in the Fraser Valley, about an hour and a half away. Any fans wanting to go to cheer on the team simply had to get permission from their last period's teacher. What Grade 8 girl wouldn't jump at the opportunity to miss last class to watch senior boys run around in shorts? Barb phoned Mom to ask for her approval, and then she called her husband to tell him she would be late coming home. I was carried onto the awaiting school bus, my wheelchair was stowed underneath. I was part of the group.

When first-term report cards were mailed out, several students, including myself, were called to the office at the end of last class. I was so embarrassed; only students in trouble were called to the office. Instead, the principal gave us a letter congratulating us for being on the Honour Roll. Great! What was the Honour Roll? Barb explained that it recognized those students with good grades. Cool. Suddenly, I was very proud of myself! Mom and Dad were proud, too. On my next day off, they splurged by rewarding my hard work with lunch at Cloud Nine, the revolving restaurant atop the Sheraton Hotel in downtown Vancouver. Very nice!

I soon realized that after being on the Honour Roll my first term of Grade 8, I had to work equally hard, if not harder, to remain there. Everyone now knew I could do it, so good grades were always *expected* from me. Being on the Honour Roll each term for the academic year entitled me, along with my family and a couple of guests, to attend the year-end Awards Ceremony, where I was presented with an Academic Award. It was a great evening. Inwardly, I didn't mind being recognized, along with the school's best students, for my hard work and accomplishment. I did receive an Academic Award for three out of the five high school grades, slightly missing the Honour Roll only a few times. I also received the Outstanding Junior Student Award in Grade 10. Not bad, considering they doubted my academic abilities prior to entering high school.

In February, I got my first electric scooter, my little Amigo. It was mainly black with a bright yellow cover over the motor, and it reminded me of a bumblebee. Mom and I had seen a woman in an Amigo at a shopping mall while we were on vacation the previous summer. The seat actually swiveled so that the woman could easily stand up at the cashier to pay for her purchases. We had never seen such a neat thing. We caught up with the woman and asked her about it. It seemed ideal for me.

When we mentioned it to my physio, she hadn't heard about it. She tried putting me in a small, low electric wheelchair. She set up an obstacle course in the therapy room and let me try it very briefly. When she saw that I wasn't steering the chair very well, she yanked me out, and that was the end of it. She even suggested to Mom that I should not have an electric wheelchair. It didn't seem to matter to her that the hand control was on the right side, and I'm left-handed! I felt like a sixteen-year-old who is given the much-anticipated, first opportunity to drive a car in a deserted parking lot and then is not allowed to drive anymore because she can't handle the car. She hasn't had any driving lessons yet!

Anyway, Mom and Dad located an Amigo scooter at a medical equipment store and arranged for me to try it for a day at school. It was wonderful! And, I think Barb enjoyed the break from pushing my wheelchair up the long ramp for the day.

Despite my physio's opinion, Mom and Dad decided to purchase the Amigo. I no longer had to rely on others to push my wheelchair. I was so excited about the freedom to go where I wanted, whenever I wanted! Driving it took some practice, and I did run over a number of toes in the process. I even had a recurring nightmare of losing control and driving down the stairs at school, particularly the open staircase in the library. Thankfully, that never happened.

One Saturday, Dad and an Industrial Arts teacher spent time in the workshop, rigging up a system so that I could carry my typewriter on the back of my scooter. It worked great, like a turtle carrying his home with him. Then a student in each class would put my typewriter up on the desk at the beginning of class and take it down at the end. Barb's job was becoming obsolete.

Shortly afterwards came another momentous day. My friend Beth lived around the corner from us, five or six houses up the street. She invited me to her house one Saturday afternoon. Mom walked with me to the corner of our short block and then watched me wheel up to my friend's house, which, luckily, had a ground-floor entrance with a family room on that level. This was the first time I was able to go to a friend's house alone, without needing a parent to drive me. I was spreading my wings! One giant leap for Glenda's independence!

My Amigo scooter not only gave me a form of independent mobility; it also gave me an independent self-identity. I no longer needed someone always around me to push my wheelchair. I no longer needed to be attached to someone or someone attached to me. I was no longer under someone's control when moving. With my Amigo, I could move around without someone behind me, towering over me. I could move independently, a whole new experience.

The Glenda-Barb team was slowly loosening. Barb began training volunteer classmates to take carbon copy notes for me. NCR (no carbon required) paper did not exist yet, so Barb had them use old-fashioned carbon paper, which Dad *obtained* from work, and a plain sheet of paper under their lined notepaper. As long as the students remembered to place the carbon paper face down it worked great. With one classmate setting up my typewriter and another one taking notes in each class, Barb gradually disappeared during class time.

Part way through the spring term, Student Council, of which I was a member throughout my high school career, organized a Spirit Week, a week of various activities held during lunch hour. One event was the Tricycle Race in which a team of three students and one teacher rode a child's trike around an obstacle course in a relay fashion. To not miss out on the fun, I put a team together, consisting of Wacky Watson, Funny Fennell, Dingbat DeBeer and (Mr.) Jazzy Janzen, and borrowed Ian's trike. Since my Amigo scooter had three wheels, it qualified as a tricycle. Mr. Janzen, our math teacher, helped me at the various checkpoints where I had to do things like eating dry crackers and then drinking lemonade. It was silly fun!

Barb stood with the other spectators, cheering us on. She had performed her job so well that, by the end of the school year, she had worked herself out of a job. I no longer needed a full-time aide. All apron strings were now cut. I was now ready to fly on my own! The following years Mom came to school with me for the first week to help set up note takers and *typewriter putter-uppers* in each class and to calm any teacher's fears. Then I was on my own. I handled nearly everything on my own. For each and every test, I arranged for the teacher to leave it with the librarian, where I would write it, and then the teacher picked it up. Some teachers quickly learned the routine; others needed constant reminders.

In Grade 12, I attended my first Friday night party at Steve's house. I was excited yet nervous. I hadn't met his parents before, and I wasn't sure how they would react to me. His dad greeted me at the door, "Hi love, come on in." No problem. Having three teenaged boys, Steve's parents knew there was no way to prevent them from partying, so they opened their family room in the basement for the weekend ritual. They figured their boys were safer partying at home than driving home drunk from somewhere, which made sense.

Steve and I sat around, joking and playing a few games of crib. Having only heard about these parties, I also did a lot of watching, taking it all in. I remember Steve commenting that I was all eyes that night. Mom had written our phone number on a piece of paper for Steve to call when I was ready for a ride home. Figuring she probably didn't want to stay up too late, I reluctantly had him call about ten. Relying on others for rides puts a damper on one's social life. Mom answered the phone, "What's the matter, Steve? Is Glenda driving up your stairs now?" Quick-witted Steve responded, "No, she's driving back down them now!" What a sense of humour!

The next week, I was doing homework on the computer set up for me in the Learning Assistance Centre. I wasn't keen on being there, as I felt like I was back in Special Ed class. Anyway, I was working, minding my own business, when an English teacher came over. She had taught my English 10 class, as well as Steve's Modified English class. She said, "I hear you were at Steve's house, playing poker. Should you really be doing that?" I have never played poker in my life; in fact, I have no clue how to play. However, at that moment, I had an urge to reply, "Yeah, strip poker…and I lost!" I would have loved to seen her reaction. Instead, I simply smiled sweetly. Occasionally, being *non-verbal* is a blessing. It has kept me out of hot water many times.

I speculated that, in her opinion, if people couldn't understand Shakespeare or diagram sentences, they weren't worthy as friends. Imagine her chagrin when I asked Steve to be my date at Grad. Not sure if there were restrictions on who could be a date for the Grad Banquet and Dance, Mom and I asked my guidance counselor if it was alright to invite someone from Grade 11. I typed an invitation for Steve, which Kevin then delivered during his weekend paper route. Steve called almost immediately to accept my invitation. Yes!

Plans were put in motion. Mom made my dress, a long, shimmering turquoise gown with a fitted bodice and short, Princess Di sleeves. My friend Shona and I booked one table together for our dates, parents, and Auntie Fern, who came over from Vancouver Island for the occasion.

May 18, 1984, finally arrived. Grade 12 students were given the day off to prepare for the evening, after receiving lectures from almost every teacher on the dangers of drinking and driving. Teachers dread that time of year. And, although it was supposedly a dry Grad, bottles were still passed under the tables. Even the vice-principal had suspiciously rosy cheeks by the end of the evening.

The event was held at the Vancouver Italian Cultural Centre, the only place large enough at that time to hold our class. After a typical buffet dinner, the obligatory speeches, and the Parade of Grads, the Dance began. The first dance was for Grads and their dates. Steve and I headed onto the dance floor; this was only my second time on the dance floor in my life, and, as the band hit the first notes, I realized it was a slow song! Great. I wondered how the heck we were going to do that. Steve asked, "Does your seat turn?" I undid the release and turned my chair. Without hesitation, he got down on one knee, put one arm around my waist, took my left hand in his, and we danced my first slow dance!

I don't know if he had laid awake nights, thinking of how he would handle such a situation, or if the idea came to him at that moment. Either way, it was definitely not something the average teenaged guy would have done! His qualities were more special than a thorough understanding of Shakespeare and grammar.

He once told Mom that he was afraid to take me on a date in case I needed to go to the washroom. Mom replied, "Don't worry. Glenda is like a camel." Thanks Mom! Looking back, it was a lot for a sixteen- or seventeen-year-old kid to consider a relationship with a girl with cp. He likely had questions unsure how to ask. Given different circumstances, Steve and I may have taken our friendship further. I give him credit for the friendship that we did have back then, something no other guy attempted in high school. It was difficult to have that perspective as a teenaged girl, especially once Steve had a girlfriend. The green monster called jealousy reared his ugly head for the first time.

After Grad, we still faced a few weeks of school and final exams. I also had to prepare for two scholarship exams as well as the provincial finals. Because of my slow typing speed using only my left thumb, we had to get special permission from the Ministry of Education for me to have three times the allotted time for writing the exams. We succeeded.

We arranged for me to write my exams in the library, as usual, and a school-appointed individual would invigilate the test and supervise any breaks I needed. Mom volunteered. She sat at the table behind me, knitting. I heard the click-clack of her needles, a sound that was comforting in a way, as I wrote the exams.

Students writing for scholarships wrote the provincial exam followed by the scholarship exam for a total of three hours. The Algebra exam was first on the schedule. Imagine using a Smith Corona typewriter to write all the steps necessary to solve Algebra problems, substituting typewritten symbols for math symbols. I was allowed up to 9 hours, if needed, and it took me 8 ¾ hours! The secretary had to stay to lock up my completed exam and the office door! I was exhausted, yet I still had to prepare for the next exam. Mom strongly recommended to the principal that I be allowed to break up the two exams into two days. He agreed, but it was still a brutal week or two.

Commencement was held the end of June. Actual diplomas weren't presented as final exams had yet to be marked. Instead rolled, blank papers were presented, and diplomas were mailed later. Imagine receiving only a blank page after all those years of work!

Due to the workload, I had decided to complete Grades 11 and 12 in three years; thus, I did not graduate with my class. This was not an easy decision, but it was realistic as my left thumb can type only so fast. Despite this, Mom and I attended the ceremony as special guests so that I could watch my friends and classmates graduate, most of whom did not know I was not graduating with them until that moment. Once everyone else had received their blank pieces of paper, the principal specially recognized me sitting in the front row. My classmates gave me a standing ovation. It was difficult to hold back the tears.

As if the first time around wasn't difficult enough, in September I went back to school with a new group of kids for Grade 12 The Sequel. I felt like I had flunked and was kept back a grade. And, to make matters worse, I took two Grade 11 courses with kids two years younger than me, which didn't do much for my self-esteem. Despite that, I did make a few friendships that still exist today; in fact, one became my roommate for one semester at university.

I did go to the Grad Banquet and Dance again – with Mom and Dad. It wasn't quite the same, especially without Steve, who went with his girlfriend. Imagine that! However, he did ask me for one dance.

As soon as final exams and year-end activities were done, we packed a moving van and headed north to the Cariboo, in the interior of British Columbia. My parents had succumbed to the 18% mortgage rates. We had to move.

Moving day was a day from hell; nothing went right. Mom and three kids drove in the van, following Dad and one brother in the moving truck. The trip, which normally took about six hours, was extraordinarily long. The truck crawled up Jack Ass Mountain, in the Fraser Canyon, at ten miles per hour. Because of a problem with our tent trailer connectors not fitting with the moving truck connectors, there were no signal and brake lights operating on the trailer, which was highly illegal. Mom had to keep right behind Dad the entire way, not letting any cars – particularly police cars – come between us. For endless hours Mom and I stared at the back of the moving truck: *U Haul – Adventures in Moving!* No kidding!

Barely unpacked, Mom and I left for Finland for nearly four weeks to attend Miilu '85, the international Girl Guide and Boy Scout camp. When we returned, we settled into country living. We rented a log house on approximately one hundred twenty acres facing Abel Lake, which was more like a pond. We were about thirty minutes from town, 100 Mile House, and could see only one neighbour from our house. This was quite a change from city life, and at times it was a cultural shock!

Commencement was held in September, which meant we actually received our diplomas! The whole family drove down for the event. Besides, we had to pick up some belongings that were stored at a friend's because they would not fit in the moving truck.

The Commencement Ceremony was nice. Because the accessible route onto the stage was lengthy and roundabout, I watched most of the evening from behind the large velvet curtain. One of the drawbacks of having a last name beginning with W is the long wait. When I finally received my certificate, the audience gave me a standing ovation. It was difficult to fight back the tears. And, as Steve received his certificate and walked off the stage, he peeked behind the curtain to give me a great big smile and a "thumbs up". I had done it! I had completed high school in a *regular* school, taking *regular* classes! It was time to move on to the next chapter and challenge in my life.

COUNTRY LIFE

Our log house was situated atop a rolling hill, with a quarter-mile driveway from the dirt road. The 120 acres was fairly open and scattered with groves of aspen trees. Down the hill from the front of the house was a small trapper's cabin. When my parents later cleaned it out to convert it into a goat barn, they found newspapers dated from the 1940s and earlier strewn about and stuffed as insulation into cracks between the logs.

Down from the cabin was the pond-sized Abel Lake. It was one of several thousand lakes that dot the rolling hills of Cariboo country, an area well travelled during the Cariboo Gold Rush, centered 185 miles north in Barkerville in the 1860s. The area is rich in history and fascinating tales of the adventures of men in search of their elusive fortunes. Since that time the Cariboo relies on cattle ranching, logging and tourism for subsistence.

In the spring, the fields around the house were golden with dandelions, seemingly more beautiful than the pesky weed variety found in manicured city lawns. In summer, gentle breezes rippled through the tall wild grasses like rolling waves on the ocean. And in the winter, which came rather early as the first snow fell in early September, the snow was covered in sparkling diamonds.

Separating the field from the house yard was a zigzagged, log fence. Rather than a gate, which would have been a nuisance opening and closing each time, there was a cattle guard at the end of the driveway. A cattle guard is a shallow trench, a few feet wide, with poles laid across and spread far enough apart so cattle could not cross yet vehicles could drive over with no problem.

For water, we relied on a well with an electric pump. This was not a problem until our first power outage, of which there were many, when we discovered that we had no water for drinking or flushing. Large, blue water jugs holding reserves for when we lost power became part of our bathroom décor. The well water turned our cooked rice a yellow-green, almost fluorescent, tinge. Mom didn't dare have the water tested since there was nothing we could really do about it anyway. She discovered that by simply adding a bit of lemon juice, the rice came out white. Sometimes it is best not to know why!

We also had a sewage lagoon, which is as it sounds and was definitely not a second pond! On a hot summer's day, when the breeze was just right, we were reminded of its existence. We were reminded again in winter when the top water froze, causing pressure to back up into the house. We learned the hard way that a hole had to be cut in the ice to release the pressure. Every subsequent winter morning, before anyone could flush, Dad had to trek to the sewage lagoon to chop a hole in the ice. A few axes and chainsaws were lost in the sludge, much to Mom's chagrin.

Once Mom and I returned from the Scouting and Guiding jamboree in Finland and Dad returned from working at a summer camp for children with learning disabilities, we settled into the novelty of country living. We had a fair bit of company in the late summer and early fall. People were curious to see where we were now living, and they wanted to make sure we would survive the winter and not drop off the face of the earth. We even took in the 100 Mile Country Harvest Fall Fair that September. I was beginning to feel I was living in Laura Ingalls' *Little House on the Prairie*.

Freed from the 18% mortgage that hung like an albatross around my parents' necks, there was a sense of relief. Laughter and fun were back in the family, at least temporarily. Mom and Dad went for walks, holding hands, and came back laughing. Even though I knew it was no longer an option, I secretly wished that a baby sister would soon be on her way; a wish I never revealed until now!

Grandma joined us for our first white Christmas in the Cariboo, which was definitely a welcomed change from the green Christmases we had down on the coast. Christmas was more joyful than it had been in the past few years, as was evident by the few more gifts under the tree. Grandma was like an excited, small child with twinkling eyes as she opened her first-ever Christmas stocking; she had never had a stocking as a child. Considering that she had always contributed white, tissue-wrapped surprises to our stockings, it was extra special to give that first to her.

Given Grandma's love of the English language, we played Dictionary while sitting around the kitchen table. She laughed and laughed at the word *titmouse*. She had such an infectious laugh. This was the second most memorable Christmas we shared together as a family, the first being the one spent at the Forbidden Plateau Lodge on Vancouver Island.

With money donated by the two local Lions Clubs, I bought my first computer, a Commodore 64, and started the Certified General Accountant (CGA) Program by correspondence in December. Having no bookkeeping experience and no access to resources beyond my textbooks, it was a challenge to learn on my own. Dad helped me where he could.

The plan, which had been briefly discussed with the guidance counsellor my final year of high school, was to become a CGA simply because I was good at math and because accounting could be completely done on computer. I would start my own business, working from home to avoid the transportation issue. That was the extent of the career planning I received in high school. Nobody cared that I didn't have a clue what accountants actually did or that I hadn't taken any bookkeeping or business courses in high school.

As I took a break from studying one day, not that there was much else for me to do, Mom hinted that I get back into my room to study. She remarked, "A lot of people are counting on you." That comment was permanently etched in my memory. I was expected to do well so as to not disappoint anyone else. I wondered where all those people were as I sat alone in my bedroom, trying to learn accounting principles and economics on my own. That remark has echoed in my head many, many times.

The morning of my first final exam, which I wrote at home with a local CGA invigilating, Dad picked up our first batch of day-old chicks from the feed store. He returned home before I began my exam. I took one look in the box and in disappointed shock, exclaimed, "They aren't yellow!" I was expecting fluffy, yellow chicks. In children's books, on television and in pictures, they were always yellow, so I assumed ALL chicks were yellow. These were black, not yellow! This city girl had a lot to learn. The chicks were to be *temporarily* in the living room under heat lamps until it was warm enough to put them in the chicken coop, so I listened to *peep peep peep* as I wrote my exam in my bedroom for 8.25 hours!

These chicks were egg layers and eventually laid beautiful, brown eggs. Our next chicks were bred to produce large amounts of meat. They put on so much weight that their poor legs couldn't support them. When we had chicken for dinner, I typically had the drumsticks because they were easy for me to pick up and eat. The leg bones were bent, and, oftentimes, broken. That combined with the stench when plucking and gutting the chickens in the kitchen is why I can't stomach gnawing on a drumstick in the style of King Henry VIII any more.

Shortly before the arrival of the chicks came the goats. Our first goat we bought came with two kids: the doeling which Ian, who was studying Egypt in school, named Hathor, the goddess of love, and the buckling, which we referred to as "Bucko" even though we were cautioned against bonding with him as he was destined for the slaughterhouse. How was I not to bond with this gorgeous creature with a shiny, sleek black coat with a tiny white dab on his forehead, so muscular and yet so gentle? The only young, strong, handsome male around for miles, he was four-legged and destined for the freezer. Just my luck!

That was a difficult concept for this animal loving, city girl to swallow. I cried for days at the thought of having to eat a friend. That was one part of country life I found very difficult. Given the choice, I would have preferred being vegetarian. But, not having that choice, I ate what was put in front of me.

Frequently, Dad drove the van down to the barn so that I could join him for the evening milking chores. We first fed the kids their bottles, with me sitting on a hay bale. Once they were all fed in turn, Dad sat me on a large plastic lid placed on the ground in the kids does' pen so that I could play with them as Dad milked the adult does. My

Nubian baby goat, with long floppy ears, appropriately named Valerie since she was born on Valentine's Day, sometimes laid down on my lap once she had her fill of hay. Dad left me down at the barn until supper was ready, and then he walked back down the hill to drive me up to the house.

The time spent with Dad at the barn was good. He and I hadn't spent an abundance of time alone together. Mom was involved with my therapy or school, while Dad was busy with Scouting activities with the three boys. We didn't talk too much at the barn because he was moving about and couldn't focus on what I was saying; the time together was nice. And, we shared that one interest – the goats.

Next came the sheep, Ian's 4H project; however, much to my disappointment there wasn't a horse in sight. Soon the animals took priority over the people. Those of us not directly involved in the livestock became somewhat invisible.

My contact with the outside world included making occasional trips to town with my parents, writing to a few friends from high school, and assisting Mom with the Brownie Pack, until the snow made it too difficult for Mom to carry my manual wheelchair and then me up the chapel stairs to where we met.

The following summer, I applied to attend the World Conference for Youth in Nanaimo on Vancouver Island. Although my uncle was organizing the event as part of his PhD thesis and sent me an information package, he had no role in the application approval process. My application had to be approved on my own merits. I was accepted!

With another participant from Williams Lake, I flew down to Vancouver and then over to Nanaimo. A conference volunteer picked us up from the airport and drove us to the hotel. As this was my first time making this kind of trip without my parents, it was somewhat scary. No one was familiar with *Glenda-ish*. Yet, in other ways it was exhilarating as I was completely on my own and totally responsible for myself. Uncle was floating around in the background, but I didn't see much of him that week as he was busy making sure the conference of several hundred youth from around the world was successful. Two volunteers were available to assist me when I did need help.

The conference sessions were about various ways young people were creating employment and making a difference, often without the aid from government-funded programs. I was exposed to interesting, new ideas from around the world, including countries I hadn't heard of before. I was also exposed to different cultures, beliefs and ways of doing things. There is richness in diversity, which is exhilarating in itself.

Time spent outside of the sessions was equally stimulating. I met Rodney from Northern Ireland who was searching for ways to bring Catholic and Protestant youths together in acceptance and understanding; we corresponded for several years afterwards. I danced with people from Pakistan, Bangladesh, Tongo and Switzerland and was amazed by the wide variety of dance styles. I was given a silver bracelet engraved in a foreign script with *Eternal Love* from a fellow from Nepal; he took the bracelet off his wrist and placed it on mine as we were dancing. I learned that Iceland allows every kind of alcohol except beer, although it's possible that Asgeir was using that as an excuse for enjoying large quantities of Canadian beer. I was carried off the boat by Steve from Switzerland when we all attended a conference-organized picnic on a nearby island.

There are some benefits to not being able to walk; I never pass up the opportunity to be carried by a handsome guy!

Late one night I watched Prince Andrew's and Lady Sarah's wedding while lying in bed, trying to keep my eyes open. Watching television with a remote control in bed was a new, luxurious experience.

Attending the conference and meeting other young people from around the world confirmed what I had been feeling for quite a while; I was missing out on life. There was much happening out there in the world, and I wasn't part of it. I really wanted to get out and experience life and explore the world. After all, I would only be young once, and "life" wasn't marching up Abel Lake Road.

Between that and reading letters from my friends at university, I began thinking about going to university; correspondence wasn't enough for me. I wanted social interaction and new ideas. Wheels started turning ever so slowly in that direction.

Adding to that frustration, Rick Hansen completed his Man in Motion Tour in May 1987. I was envious of his wheeling around the world, seeing so many countries and meeting people from such diverse cultures. And, in my naïve mind, I thought the only real difference in our abilities and disabilities was his normal speech. Except for that, why couldn't I do something amazing like he had done, rather than simply sitting in the country? My hunger grew more intense.

At the official closing to Rick's journey, our Premier announced he would establish a Premier's Advisory Committee to examine the barriers facing British Columbians with disabilities. Eager to participate, I wrote a letter to the Premier, expressing my interest in being involved with such a committee. A few weeks later, Dad answered the phone. To his surprise it was someone from the Premier's Office, saying that my letter had been received and that someone would be in touch later. Although I don't think that second phone call ever came, it indicated to me that, with a higher education and more experience, I had the potential to meet with influential people, to affect change.

Having graduated from high school, Kevin left for Banff, Alberta on Canada Day 1987. He had a job as a dishwasher at the world-famous Banff Springs Hotel. He went to experience another corner of Canada and to save for university in September. He found his niche in the world, thoroughly enjoying the Banff area in the Rocky Mountains. His plans changed, and he put university on hold. He still lives in the Banff area today.

Mom also left that summer to attend summer school at the University of British Columbia. Between raising four kids and working full-time for most of those years, she was still trying to complete her Bachelor of Education. Now living so far from civilization and the university campus, going for intensive courses during the summer months was Mom's only opportunity for completing her degree.

The house was quiet that summer, and it was strange without Mom. I had to survive on the strange cooking of my Dad and brothers. Our sheltie dog Bonnie became much weaker that summer, barely able to stand. One afternoon in late August she was lying on the kitchen floor, and it was obvious the end was near. Neal, Dad and I were the only ones home at the time, and for some reason we were all around the kitchen at that particular moment. We stood there, watching, not sure what to do. At the end, Dad grabbed a garbage bag and knelt down beside her. I saw him cry for only the second time in my life, as he picked up

Bonnie and carried her outside. Although I never asked and Dad never said, I know he took her to the insinuator, the 40-gallon barrel used for burning garbage. It seemed like an unfit way to say goodbye to a dear friend, but that is how things are done in the country.

Bonnie had been a part of our family for more than sixteen years. We had picked her from a litter at the breeder's kennel. I remember getting to choose her name; I had the choice between *Honey* and *Bonnie*. Sitting down on the kennel floor with puppies jumping and bouncing all over me, loving every moment of it, I chose Bonnie because it was easier to say.

Next came housebreaking and obedience training. We entered Bonnie in several dog shows. Spending a day in an arena full of dogs was heaven to me. According to Dad, I had the ability to pick the winners before the judges announced them. I saved every one of Bonnie's ribbons in an empty Kleenex box.

When it came time to have her bred for the first time, we took her to another breeder that ours had recommended. There were many tears as we left her for a few days. Shortly afterwards, a frantic breeder called to say Bonnie had escaped from the kennel and could not be found. I remember all of us driving there after school, waiting in the car until way past dark as Mom and Dad called and searched for Bonnie to no avail. In the end, they left a pair of my pants in a nearby shed in hopes that she would smell them and curl up with them until morning. Being a rural, farming area, there was a danger of coyotes, and Bonnie wouldn't stand a chance against them. We drove home in silence.

The next morning, this heartbroken six-year-old bravely told her teacher the news. There was great relief and joy when Dad brought Bonnie to school later in the day. A nearby farmer had spotted her and lured her into a barn with a ham bone until Dad could arrive to pick her up. With me hugging her for dear life and her wagging her tail wildly, I don't know who was more excited, Bonnie or me. She was definitely this human's best friend!

A couple of months later, Neal went running to Mom, excitedly yelling, "'Mommy, Bonnie pooped a puppy! Bonnie pooped a puppy!" And so began our years of Sheltie puppies and dogs everywhere. To this day, I have a soft spot for sable-coloured Shetland sheepdogs, miniature Lassies.

In the summer of 1987, the Abel Lake property was put on the market by the owner and, as my parents had no intentions of purchasing it, they figured it was best to move before potential buyers began streaming through our home. We moved to a house on a piece of land that friends had acquired solely for the hay fields at Fawn Lake, southeast of 100 Mile House. The place was a better arrangement for the animals. There were a few more sheds, properly fenced corrals suitable for the goats, sheep, and soon-to-be-acquired steer, and actual livestock waterers that would save Dad and Ian from lugging water buckets a few times a day.

Even though it was a good move for the livestock, it wasn't as great for the humans. The house was much smaller than the one at Abel Lake; in fact, it was claustrophobic at times. For me, I had no way of getting outside on my own as there were stairs at both the front and back doors. The promised ramp never materialized.

Tension between my parents began escalating. An awkward silence was settling in the house, except for the frequent slamming of doors. I began missing the doorless kitchen cupboards in the Abel Lake house. The idyllic adventure in country living had become a less than desirable situation. Cracks in the family were beginning to appear. Although I was scared, it was time to leave the crumbling family nest and to experience new adventures.

Atop the Hill

New Year's Day morning, 1988, in -35°C temperatures, Mom and Ian stuffed my bed frame (minus the foam mattress), our old arborite kitchen table, my new microwave, my Commodore 64 computer, my clothes and other belongings into the Beaumont car, and then the three of us crammed into the front seat. I was off to university!

I was excited yet terrified at the same time. I had been having chest pains for a few months, which intensified as New Year's Day neared. Amazingly, they disappeared once I arrived and settled into university life.

When I initially started talking about going to university, Mom was thinking I meant the following September, giving us plenty of time to organize details. Even though I had been accepted into Simon Fraser University without a problem, the apparent wait was going to be for housing, which was very limited. Much to our amazement, a one-bedroom apartment came available for January. It was mine if I wanted it, so I jumped at the opportunity.

Plans were put into fast forward. Auntie Fern and her then partner scrounged some used furniture from a motel they were redecorating. The apartment quickly became home, furnished in the eclectic look – very cozy, yet bright as the place faced due south. Living above the garbage room, a definite *fragrance* wafted in all summer, and it wasn't relaxing aromatherapy! I was directly across from another residence, so I could watch my neighbours as clearly as they could watch me. Living in a fishbowl took some getting used to after living in the country. Although, this proximity proved to be handy when my TV's picture died; I listened to mine and watched one across the way!

Mom had to return home for work within a day or two of driving me down, but Ian stayed with me for a few days to help me organize my classes, buy my books, and set up my life in a strange, new place. I was scared when he left. I felt so alone that I cried while my roommate Barb drove him to the bus station.

Being in a new place where I didn't know which way was up, and where nobody understood *Glenda-ish* was a little overwhelming. My main form of communication was by notes I had typed beforehand, trying to anticipate all the information that would be needed in that particular *conversation*. This took some planning and forethought! I went through several dozen pads of Post-It notes during my university years. I dubbed them my *talking papers*.

The first week of my first semester was somewhat intimidating. I planned to *ask* someone in each of my classes to take carbon copy notes for me as I had during high school. The critical difference was that Mom wasn't at university like she had been in high school, acting as my mouth to ask for me. This time, I essentially shoved notes in strangers' faces, asking if they would be willing to take carbon copy notes. I didn't need anything fancy or special; they simply would give me whatever notes they took for themselves, and I would fill any gaps when I listened to the lecture tapes that I had arranged for the Audio-Visual Centre to record for me. I listened to most lectures twice, once live and once taped. Now that was a dedicated student!

The task of finding note-takers wasn't easy for me. It took a fair bit of tenacity, and it didn't get easier over the years. In fact, there were some odd courses in which I never asked anyone to take notes for me. Instead, I took notes solely from the tapes, which took an inordinate amount of time. However, most people who I did *ask* were willing to do it and were nice about it. In a couple of courses, the professors gave me copies of their lecture notes along with strict orders not to pass them around to other students. I respected and honoured their trust in me.

In addition to adjusting to university life, Barb and I had the challenge of learning to live together. We had been lab partners in Biology 11 during my Grade 12 The Sequel year of high school, and we began corresponding by letters once I moved to the country. She even came up to visit one Spring Break. However, we didn't know each other that well until we became roommates.

You don't really know someone until you live together, and we definitely learned a lot about each other that semester! It was a strain at times. Because I needed her help with some things, I felt like I couldn't say what was bothering me about other things in case she stopped helping me. No doubt, she felt extra pressure to help me and to do more than half of the cooking and cleaning.

Despite that, Barb and I became best of friends and had numerous good times together. One involved the two of us, her cousin, my Amigo scooter and a 10-speed bike all crammed into her Volkswagen Bug! Mysteriously, the piece of Black Forest cake was never found! Hmmm.

We made several trips to Barb's home to do laundry and to enjoy her mom's cooking. Her family became like a second family to me, even after she left to study in Germany and, subsequently, met her husband. It was comforting knowing I had people there who I could count on; and I did, sometimes for the strangest things! When she moved back home after that first semester, we agreed to remain friends. After all, we had too much dirt on one another to be anything else! We are still friends today, although, unfortunately, we're not as close.

The main reason I chose Simon Fraser University over the University of British Columbia, which would have been my first preference based on the character of the campus and the number of services and things to do on campus, was because it was more wheelchair accessible at that time. Situated atop Burnaby Mountain, the SFU campus was then fairly compact. When the campus was built in the 1960s, wheelchair accessibility was at least considered in most areas, although it often involved taking a roundabout route to navigate the cement jungle.

I saw parts of campus that most students did not know even existed. At those moments, particularly when it was rainy and foggy like gray, pea soup, I would curse the architect, thinking, "If I ever meet him in a dark alley…" The worst was a ramp nicknamed Suicide Hill. It was so steep! I literally had to pull my little Amigo scooter up the ramp by grabbing the handrail with one hand and steering with the other. Rumour had it that Rick Hansen trained on it prior to his Man in Motion World Tour because it was the steepest incline in the area.

One day when heading down this long, steep ramp, I hit a wet patch, no doubt from yet another crack in the cement, and lost control! As my scooter was building frightening speed, I was scared that if I didn't miraculously stop, I would crash head on into the cement wall at the bottom of the ramp; an outcome I didn't want to imagine. Thankfully, my dual back wheels caught the post of the handrail, suddenly stopping my runaway scooter. The only damage was a slightly bent axel, which Facilities Management fixed for me.

Another time I was heading up the ramp after a Psychology tutorial, and the belt on my scooter broke. In that very instant, I realized the critical role of the belt! I had no power and no control, and I was rapidly rolling backwards down the hill! Luckily, the scooter turned and tipped. Again, I narrowly missed colliding with that cement wall, although it did give me more nightmares.

My teaching assistant was heading back to her office and saw me in a crumpled heap on the ramp. She righted my scooter and then helped me back into it. As I already had a goose egg forming on my head, she insisted on taking me to Health Services; she pushed my scooter as I steered. Although I had no broken bones, I had a mild concussion and several bruises, which turned colourful over the next few days. Once the doctor finished examining me and writing a complete incident report, this sweet TA pushed me back to residence and made sure someone would check on me in a couple of hours. Amazingly, there was always someone around when I really needed help, and I truly appreciated each one. I spent that weekend at Barb's house, soaking up some special attention, while her dad repaired my scooter.

My parents probably cringed every time I called with such horror stories. Being six hours away, there wasn't much they could do. I knew if it were really serious, they would be there; in fact, Mom once made the trip simply to take me grocery shopping. I could ask my friends only so many times to help me. That was before the public buses were wheelchair accessible, so I was literally stuck atop the hill, sometimes for eight or nine weeks at a time, at which point I started going stir crazy!

Somewhere along the line, I reconnected with my godfather / proxy uncle and aunt. They often picked me up for Sunday dinner with them, their four grown kids and significant others. I became part of the family. They would also take me to various events around town, which gave me much-appreciated breaks from campus and never-ending homework. They became a significant support in my life, for which I am sincerely grateful.

Once Barb moved out, I tried doing everything myself: the laundry, the cooking and the cleaning. But, with no grocery store on campus and no way of me getting off the hill myself, I had to rely on my two friends with cars to take me grocery shopping. That dependency wasn't good for our friendships. I also had no way of having a bath independently. After hesitating for a couple of months, I reluctantly arranged for a homemaker. The girl across the hall suggested it; she also had a physical disability and had a homemaker come in weekly to assist with the basics.

The most difficult thing was having the homemaker assist me into the tub for my weekly bath. During that time it was as if I wasn't in my own body, like I was watching from above or something. Disassociation helped me to endure the embarrassment and indignity of stripping for a total stranger during my bath, something I never shared with my *normal* friends. This was another instance where I kept separate my abled and disabled worlds.

In addition, I endured some appalling behaviour by incompetent homemakers, including being dropped in the tub and being inappropriately touched. One of them ate my food and swiped my laundry money for her bus fare, and two of them pooped on my bathroom floor. Since these were the days before most people had email and I couldn't phone the supervisor to report such misconduct – not that I felt a non-verbal disabled girl would be believed over a paid employee – I tolerated these homemakers and dreaded Thursday mornings. I figured that I had to put up with that *stuff* since I needed help. Of course, there were a few good homemakers who I looked forward to seeing each week; unfortunately, they never lasted long, moving on to more favourable and financially rewarding jobs.

I experienced several firsts while at university. One Sunday in July 1989, I went to my first rock concert! Rod Stewart. I felt like a silly teenager! I had *discovered* him a few months previously while watching the American Music Awards. I felt like a late bloomer, but I was raised on country music. I had heard some of Rod's hits, like *Maggie May* and *Tonight's the Night*, but I had never seen the man behind the raspy voice. Once I did, he became the fodder for many a fantasy!

Doing some research on Rod Stewart that summer, which gave me great practice using the library equipment while it was quiet, I discovered that his father and my grandfather were born two years apart in Edinburgh. I like to think there was a connection between the Stewarts and Marshalls and that they at least knew of each other. After all, how large was Edinburgh at the turn of the twentieth century?

One of Rod's lesser-known songs, *Never Give Up On a Dream,* helped me through many rough days. It was his tribute to Terry Fox, the Canadian who ran the Marathon of Hope to raise research funds to find a cure for cancer. After a difficult class or a frustrating situation of being *non-verbal* in a verbal world, I would go home and play that song, sometimes two or three times.

To attend one particular class, I had to go outside, around the building to a back door, which a classmate or security guard had to open from the inside. I then had to go across the lecture platform of one theatre, through a storage room with strange looking equipment, to the very front of our lecture theatre. I parked in the corner in front of the first row of seats and hoped I didn't trip the professor while he was lecturing.

Leaving the class after the lecture was also interesting. The class next door went longer than ours, and, although I was told it was alright to cut through, there was no way I wanted to scoot across the stage while that professor was still lecturing. I sat for half an hour in the storage room until that class was over. If anything had happened while I sat in that strange room, I wouldn't have been found for days. I then went to Audio-Visual to pick up my lectures tapes to begin the onerous task of listening to the lecture again to fill in any gaps or clarify any points in my classmate's notes. On days like those I listened to *Never Give Up On a Dream*, sometimes repeatedly, before I returned to the necessary state of mind. Rod Stewart still holds a majority share in my music collection.

For one Psychology course, I had to conduct an experiment that was both properly and ethically designed. After thinking about how I would run an experiment and talking with a friend who was a Kinesiology grad student, I decided to explore the strange phenomenon that able-bodied people (ABs) tend to walk straight into people in wheelchairs and then claim to have not seen the chairs. How big must a wheelchair be in order to be seen?

I designed an experiment to test my hypothesis that objects need to be at ABs' eye level to be seen. I sat in my scooter in the middle of the busy concourse during the break between classes. Twice I had a helium-filled balloon tied at eye level to my scooter; twice I did not. My Kines friend counted how many people tripped over my scooter. I don't recall whether the difference was statistically significant, but fewer people did trip when I had a balloon tied to my chair. The bottom line is ABs typically don't watch where they are walking. Yet they have driver's licenses. Yikes! I wonder if the wheelchair parking signs placed on posts are more effective than those painted on the pavement.

    Most assignments weren't that fun though. They were actually quite solitary, and I spent hours and days alone in my apartment, working on papers. I was relieved when long weekends were over and classes resumed so that I could be with people, even if it was in a non-verbal, observatory role. Strangely, I met most of my friends at Thursdays' Pub Nights, not in class. Is there anything wrong with that picture?

    Once springtime rolled around atop the hill and winter clothing was shed, I remember going about campus, observing sights of the male variety and thinking, "Woowee! Where were you hibernating all winter?" They unknowingly became material for great fantasies. A recurring one involved me jumping in my boyfriend's red convertible, tossing my manual wheelchair into the back seat, and driving down the west coast – Washington, Oregon, California. We explored quaint eateries and little shops, spent nights at out-of-the-way Bed and Breakfasts, and stopped at remote beaches to do whatever came naturally. In reality, I didn't even get to first base. Hell, I don't think I was even in the ballpark at times, and that wasn't due to a lack of interest or desire on my part!

One day I met my best friend for lunch. She was aglow as she told me about her latest romantic rendezvous the night before. I listened supportively. Then I excitedly told her about one of my guy friends, describing how I enjoyed spending time with him and how we seemed to be on the same wavelength. I always had a sense when I was about to see him, either around campus or coming by my apartment. I thought I was falling for him. She responded by saying that he didn't think of me *that* way. Once again, *that* was not meant for me. We changed the topic of conversation; he eventually married someone else.

During the summer of 1993, I did have one relationship; an online affair with a married man who was a business professor at an American university. I learned a fair bit in those few weeks! This was before the advent of chat rooms and instant messaging; in fact, I was still using Unix or Pine for email. We would be online for hours, zapping emails back and forth. Because my connection to the Internet was dialup, my aunt once tried for hours to call me and kept getting a busy signal. Eventually, she had the telephone operator interrupt the call to make sure that I was alright.

The experience was bizarre and warped for this naïve, inexperienced girl. He had an open marriage, a foreign concept to me, partly because his wife had discovered she was bisexual. They both had encounters outside of the marriage. When she flew off to be with a new man, his only concern was that the other guy might be bigger than him. I didn't understand why he wasn't worried that the guy might be an axe-murderer or be HIV-positive. It was not the healthiest situation to have as my first relationship, although that situation could never be considered healthy.

Even though we never met in person, which I definitely do not regret in the least, the experience was quite intense, with many of the emotions of a *real* relationship. It did allow me to explore my sexuality and sexual side, as our emails were very explicit at times. I soon learned not to check my email in the computer lab prior to class; otherwise, I was flushed and distracted throughout the lecture. Perhaps my preoccupation was why I only got thirty-some percent on my Child Psychology midterm. Surprisingly, and thankfully, that was actually a passing grade!

I had never had such a low grade in my life. The fact that I had been kept awake the night before by large, noisy trucks and trailers contributed to my low grade. That was my story! They were setting up an on-location movie base in our tennis courts in order to use our pool for the extremely brief water scene in the movie *Intersection*. Although exciting, the timing didn't allow me to gawk before picking up my exam. Once I returned it, however, I had time to watch from a distance and eventually saw Richard Gere shooting hoops. My first movie star sighting! I was so excited! I rushed home and phoned a couple of friends.

My steamy, email affair with the professor was short-lived. He said something that cut me to my core, which indicated to me that he didn't understand or sincerely care about me; that he was after only one thing. Although I felt physically ill when I knew the end was inevitable, once the relationship did end I felt relieved and proud of myself for standing firm for what I believed in, even if it took me a while to figure that out.

Although I wouldn't recommend it to others, I don't completely regret this bizarre encounter. It gave me the opportunity to explore, in a somewhat safe manner, a part of myself that I had no opportunity to explore previously. However, because of its secretive nature, it reinforced the message I had been receiving since Grade 5 that sexuality and sex were not for me. Any sexual interest or behaviour on my part had to be kept secret, hidden. In one letter, too late after the fact, a male friend wrote, "I made a conscious effort to keep our relationship platonic." Well, dang, Dan! Here I thought my female charms were faulty or that I was misusing them or something.

A couple years into my university career, my parents separated. I had seen it coming for a few years, although I was hoping they would work things out. I didn't want to become another dysfunctional family, another statistic. However, maybe we were already dysfunctional. Going home during semester breaks was not fun. The atmosphere was tense and strained; even Christmases were no longer joyous. I was once tempted to have a friend write *UN Peacekeeper* on a white t-shirt for me to wear home, but I decided against it.

I'm unsure what really caused the split, but years later in a moment of clarity the reasons struck me: a lack of effective communication and negotiation skills. My parents would likely say the reason was more complex, but that is how I rationalized it. Whatever the reason, it was still a very difficult time. Being created half from my Mom and half from my Dad, each battle between them felt like a war inside me. I felt like I was being torn in two as each side, overtly or covertly, expected my loyalty.

In one of my Psychology courses, we learned about family system dynamics and how one child often becomes *sick* in attempts to keep the family together. The parents focus on getting the child healthy again rather than on the marital problems. This dynamic struck a chord with me, and I thought it might be one way I could try to keep my parents together. I didn't want divorced parents and all the baggage that went with it, so here was my chance to save their marriage. I even had an illness in mind.

My Psych friend was specializing in eating disorders at that time and occasionally teased me about being anorexic because I was so skinny. Since I already looked the part, I thought I would become the part. How difficult would it be for them to believe I was actually anorexic? Not having to cook would save time and money. Then I realized that *being* anorexic meant not eating or eating very little, and I didn't know how I would do that. Although I was skinny, it was not due to not eating.

In the end, I realized it wasn't up to me to save my parents' marriage. Although I didn't understand it and had the urge to knock their heads together at times, it wasn't my place. Whatever they were going to do was their choice. However, my three brothers and I were left to deal with *our new way of life*, even though we had no say in it. Strangely, the four of us never discussed our parents' divorce and how it affected us. I dealt with it alone, in silence.

A few years into my time on the hill, a group of students with disabilities began organizing a Disabled Student Association. I went to a couple of the meetings and one of their Pizza n Movie nights, but it wasn't right for me. I was too busy being a student – researching endless papers, writing exams, watching basketball games, going to Movie Nights with friends, and, of course, the weekly Pub Night, receiving the nickname Motorcycle Mama somewhere along the way – to sit around discussing what to call ourselves: *differently abled, challenged, disAbled* and umpteen other proposed terms. I appreciated the freedom we, as people with disabilities, now had to decide how to label ourselves, but if we came up with a name too obscure, nobody would know what our group was about when looking through a list of clubs. How would new students with disabilities find us? No, it wasn't the right group for me.

Around that time, I was called into the Disabled Student Services office, which, at that time, was the assistant to the Director of Student Services helping students with disabilities off the side of her desk. Up until that point, I had only used the staff person as a resource whenever I had questions with which I thought she could help. Otherwise, I dealt directly with my professors and teaching assistants to arrange exams and other details as I had done in high school. I felt it was better to ask directly for whatever accommodations I needed rather than have someone else arrange them for me. Once I got out into the *real* world and the workplace, I would be responsible for myself and for asking and advocating for whatever special adaptations or equipment I needed. Why not do the same in university? It was my method of operating: I'll do it myself!

However, as the staff person assisting students with disabilities increased to a more full-time position, students were *encouraged* to arrange accommodations through her office. I was called in to arrange for note-takers in my classes. She arranged to have the professors announce on the first day of class that a student with a disability needed a note-taker (all eyes then turned towards me) and that interested students should go see her. The student was supplied with No Carbon Required (NCR) lined notepaper, which was easier to use than my *old-fashioned* carbon paper, and arrangements were made to have the student be paid through the Work Study Program, which was about the only real benefit to the whole process. The students that I had asked with my *talking papers* didn't seem to mind taking my notes for nothing in return. Sometimes people simply like doing a good deed to help someone else, and I didn't get the sense that they saw it as a major imposition.

As I was nearing the end of my degree, there was a trend toward requiring documentation from students with disabilities to support their requests for accommodations. Documentation was to be provided by a medical doctor or a psychologist. This need for documentation to prove the existence of a disability and the need for accommodation perpetuated the medical model of disability. My family doctor, which was the Student Health Services, was unlikely to have any clue what accommodations I required in the classroom unless I told him or her. It definitely would not have been the first time I told a doctor what to write on a medical form! Thankfully, I graduated before I was required to document my disability.

I have never fit the *disabled person* mould. Some may say I'm too independent or too stubborn, but I'm content doing things my way rather than following the path laid out for *disabled people*. I knew some students with physical disabilities who had their education paid for by Vocational Rehabilitation Services or a similar organization, which meant they had to go through a whole battery of tests and assessments to determine whether they were suitable for university and, if so, which field they should pursue. For the most part, they couldn't take a particular course unless it happened to be in their approved education plan. And they had to maintain a certain grade point average to keep their funding.

Friends who were able to pay their own way through university by flipping burgers, waiting tables or pumping gas had much more freedom in the courses they could take, even if it was only for personal interest. They could also change their major or minor several times, as long as they met the required prerequisites. To me, that personal exploration and development were as equally important as the university degree. I didn't have the time or opportunity to work my way through school since my schoolwork took most of my time and energy. And I sure didn't want to go through all that testing like I did back in Grade 7 to be told what courses I could and could not take. Forget that nonsense!

I found another way to pay for my education. Each and every semester of the seven years that I was atop the hill, I applied for bursaries, and every semester but the first one, I received one. I'm sure I had an angel looking out for me in the Financial Aid Office because sometimes I received the strangest bursaries. I was appreciative of each one as it was enough to pay my fees and books for one semester, which meant I could get one step closer to finishing my degree. I wrote a thank you note for every bursary received. In the early years, I also received the occasional open scholarship for high grades. It was like being on the Honour Roll in high school, but with money attached. Unfortunately, the university changed the rules at one point, increasing the number of credit hours to be eligible. I couldn't physically handle that many courses per semester, so that financial source disappeared. I relied on the bursaries to get me through. Thank you, my angel, whoever you were!

My final semester in spring 1995 was one of mixed emotions. I was excited to be nearly finished with my degree. It had been a very long haul, and I was ready to move on to the next chapter of my life; however, the unknown and uncertainty were terrifying. Also weighing on my mind was Convocation Day. After watching all my friends graduate and leave, my turn had come at last! But graduating meant both parents would be there, hopefully, and I knew it would be difficult and uncomfortable for them to be in close proximity. I seriously considered intentionally failing a course to avoid graduating. Perhaps I could become involved in another e-affair! Instead, I did my best and graduated with a 3.64 grade point average! Not bad for someone who was, according to the *experts*, mentally retarded and should have been institutionalized.

The uncertainty of what came next and where I would live was scary. My aunt and uncle had taken me around various areas the previous semester to see where several co-operative and subsidized housing options were located and to get a sense of them. They pointed out which areas were acceptable and which should be avoided. I applied to a couple of co-ops and to BC Housing early in my final semester, but I didn't hear anything until it was getting down to nail-biting time. On April 1st I went to look at a wheelchair-accessible unit, which was a rarity in the Vancouver area, available through BC Housing. It was a nice, clean complex on a now-accessible bus route. I decided to take it because I didn't know if I would find another accessible unit in time. In between studying for my last set of final exams, I packed boxes. I moved in at the end of the month.

By the time I left SFU after seven years, I had spent a quarter of my life at university! It had become my first home away from home. SFU was more than a place of higher education for me. It was my community, my world. I felt safe there, and I knew what areas to avoid. More importantly, I knew what was expected, and I could successfully meet those expectations. It was difficult for me to close my apartment door for the last time and to drive away to the unknown, with unknown expectations.

A beautiful day in June, I returned for the day. It was finally *my* day. The Convocation Mall dressed in its blue and red pomp and pageantry was for me as well as a thousand fellow graduates. The SFU convocation procession began three floors above, crossing the Reflection Pond and streaming down the stairs, then crossing the Convocation Mall to the seated area set up for the day.

Students in wheelchairs typically relinquished participating in the procession and sat in the front row, watching the procession go by like the rest of the viewing audience. Not being the typical student with a disability, I was not content with that alternative. I had worked hard, like everyone else, and I wanted my opportunity to *walk on the* water like my fellow graduands. And so I did! I lined up with the rest of them and crossed the pond with them to the top of the stairs. I then made a beeline to the elevator, along two hallways, down another elevator and out to the Convocation Mall, where I took my place in the front row next to the ramp going onto the stage.

After many speeches and many, many names called, it was finally my turn! Scooting up the ramp and hearing my name called, I suddenly choked up. The realization hit me. *I had done it! I had earned my degree! I was now a university graduate!* As I followed the stream of newly pinned alumni off the stage and along the route through the audience, I had a silly *I-did-it* grin across my face. From somewhere along the way, Mom yelled, "Yeah! Way to go, Glenda!"

I now had my Bachelor of Arts degree, with a major in Psychology and a minor in Communications. My next challenge was to figure out how to put it to use!

THE POWER OF ONE

Upon graduating from SFU, I moved into a subsidized housing complex, mainly for seniors, with a few wheelchair accessible units. I don't know why the government always lumps those two groups together, but it was quite a change of pace going from a university residence to an old folks' home. Secretly, I promised myself to be on my feet financially and in a "real" apartment within a maximum of five years.

That summer, I was busy researching, writing and organizing "A Spanner in the Works: Bridging Barriers with People with Disabilities," the first-ever workshop at SFU for teaching assistants and faculty members to promote an increased awareness and understanding about students with disabilities. Included in the preparation was the creation of a short video, showing the barriers to physical access around campus, which was an interesting experience. I would welcome the opportunity to create more videos.

The workshop was a success. And, I made a whopping $600 for approximately 200 hours of work. It was a start! The following week, I met with the head of facilities management. He was interested in a similar workshop for his staff to make them more aware of the physical barriers facing students with disabilities. I was on a roll. Perhaps my idea of an awareness consulting business had potential.

Unbeknownst to me, the Coordinator of Disabled Student Services had been also invited to the meeting. She promptly announced that they were in the process of creating a new position and that one responsibility would be conducting awareness training around campus. The meeting was over. The ball that I had started rolling had been snatched from me.

Since that door had been slammed shut, I was back to the drawing board, trying to build a business with no contacts or to find a job with no real work experience. Neither seemed very promising. Most entry-level positions require answering phones and typing at a speed of sixty words per minute, and neither is possible for a *non-verbal*, one-thumb typist.

I kept trying, getting nowhere. I found myself staying up later, doing needlework and watching television, and then sleeping in later and later. The later I slept, the guiltier I felt. I was wasting my time by being unproductive, but I didn't know what to do. Employers weren't willing to take a risk by hiring, or even interviewing, someone with such a physical disability. I was lost, and the fog was rolling in.

During this time, I became friends with Annie from down the hall. Annie was a few years younger than I and had a rare, degenerative disease. Soon she began attending an employment program for people with disabilities at the Neil Squire Foundation. She would come over some evenings to use my computer to do her homework. She suggested that I contact the program manager for assistance and handed me his business card.

Figuring I had nothing to lose, I emailed him. We arranged a meeting, during which he somewhat convinced me to apply for the Creative Employment Options (CEO) program that would be starting again in January. I was reluctant. I had always avoided programs specifically for people with disabilities; they rubbed against my grain. And,

I was worried about getting sucked into the system that I had so carefully avoided. But, at this point, I had nothing better to do. Although the prospect of going back to "school" after seven years of university didn't thrill me in the least, I decided to try it until something better came along.

For Christmas, Mom surprised me with a trip to Hawaii. She may have understood my despair and figured I needed a change of scenery, or she may have needed a break from the Cariboo cold and snow. Either way, I didn't argue. I simply packed my one bag and gathered up whatever cash I had, as we were going to share the expenses once we were there. The sun, sand, and surfers in Speedos did wonders for my spirit. Mom and I had a great time. And, except for the major heartbreak at the missed opportunity for romance with a particular surfing dude, I came home feeling renewed and optimistic.

I started the CEO Program with a sunburn and my mind still in Honolulu (and on that one surfing dude), which didn't help to encourage willing participation on my part. A few weeks into the program I sensed that I would get from the program whatever I put into it. At that point, I decided to jump right in and to gain whatever I could from the opportunity, although I still begrudged the *group therapy* feel in portions of the course. Soon the staff was scrambling to find work to keep me busy and challenged.

Part way through the program, I was strongly *encouraged* to become a client of Vocational Rehabilitation Services (VRS). They might pay for any special equipment or modifications needed at the workplace once I found a job. Then somehow Adult Services of Special Educational Technology – BC (SET BC) came into the picture, as did IAM CARES, another agency to assist people with disabilities in finding employment. CEO, VRS, SET-BC, IAM CARES – Mom and I referred to it as alphabet soup.

As I had feared, I was getting sucked deeper and deeper into the system, and I was beginning to lose a sense of control over my life. However, I did my best to hang on. At one point, I told SET-BC, "Thanks, but no thanks." The CEO staff was shocked. Apparently, clients don't say "no" to SET-BC.

SET-BC wanted to assess me for some kind of communication device that I could use during job interviews. I said that a laptop would be much more practical and versatile; I could use it at interviews, at meetings, and at the library for taking notes for my job search. SET-BC wouldn't consider it. It was rumored that, somewhere in the policy manual, it stated clients with cerebral palsy were not to receive laptops because these clients may drop and break them. This is one example of the countless, ridiculous rules, based on over-generalizations about disability, created by policymakers who have minimal understanding of living daily life with a disability. I simply said, "No, thanks." Besides, my trusty, low-tech alphabet card was less cumbersome, less intimidating to prospective employers, and worked fine.

Another thing that bothered me about the assessment process is that an *expert*, who does not know me, spends an hour or two with me. Based on that one point in time and that particular situation, this *expert* decides what would work best for me across time and in various situations. I think not. Besides, whenever going through an assessment, I feel like I give a piece of myself that I can never get back. And, with SET-BC, I felt the price was too high to pay, and I wasn't willing to pay it.

After four months, the CEO program was nearing an end. Strangely, I was not ready to leave. I had a strong sense that I was in the midst of a personal growth spurt. If I left now, I would miss the opportunity for that growth. So, I offered to be the volunteer teaching assistant for the next group. And guess who was in the next group? Thanks to Annie from down the hall who put me in touch with the Neil Squire Foundation, I met my future husband, Darrell! The seemingly small, insignificant action of one individual can have such an impact on another's life. That is the amazing power of one! Thanks, Annie.

Meet Your Mentor

While volunteering as the teaching assistant for the summer group of CEO, I also searched for employment using my newly acquired job search and cover letter-writing skills. Once I found postings for jobs I thought I could actually do, which seemed rather sparse, I had a fairly high response rate. I don't know if it was beginner's luck or if I had discovered the trick to writing those dreaded cover letters. When I did get an interview, it was difficult. I would come face-to-face with an individual or, worst yet, a panel of interviewers who were unfamiliar with *Glenda-ish* and not sure what to make of my shaky, jerky movements.

At one point, I applied for a part-time position as a newsletter coordinator. I did everything I was supposed to do, including going to the public library to research the organization and sweating over the cover letter. I was called for an interview. However, when the interviewer learned I was in a wheelchair, he refused to interview me. The office was on the second floor of a building with no elevator. The Foundation's manager suggested that he interview me in an accessible location to determine if I was a qualified candidate; if so, then the accessibility issues could be addressed or other possible solutions, such as telecommuting, could be explored. With a job offer on the table, Vocational Rehab Services would have paid for workplace accommodations, such as a stair-climber. Unfortunately, the interviewer refused to meet me elsewhere to see what kind of person I was and to see if I was capable of doing the job. He missed out on the most creative and meticulously edited newsletters ever produced by his organization.

    I was mad and hurt. I was not given the opportunity to prove what I *could* do. I definitely felt discriminated against, and I considered taking it to the Human Rights Commission. But, because it was only a part-time summer job, I didn't know if the battle would be worth the fight. I chalked it up to learning one of those tough lessons – always check the physical access of a job posting before applying. This narrowed my opportunities even further.

    Employers' fears about my assumed disability, rather than my actual disability, were keeping me from finding a job. I worked hard for seven years at university, getting myself a good education, which I was led to believe would open opportunities for me. Yet employers wouldn't give me a chance. I had a vocational counselor, an employment placement worker, a VRS worker and countless others because I was the one with the *disability*. It amazed me how many people had jobs because I was looking for work. The real barrier, in my opinion, was employers' attitudes and misconceptions about my disability. An attitude adjustment would have accomplished so much.

    With each job for which I applied, I mentally envisioned myself working in that position, whether it was a part-time newsletter coordinator for an early childhood education organization, a resource coordinator for a mental health agency, or some kind of entry-level position in the long-term disability insurance department of a national insurance company. After applying and mentally preparing for so many jobs, each one somewhat different, I didn't know whether I was coming or going. Because job opportunities for me were limited, I felt like I had to follow any opportunity that came along, which meant being flexible enough to go in any direction. In the process, I felt like I was blowing in the breeze, never sure where I'd be going next. I couldn't really focus on any one career direction, which was rather disconcerting.

Finally, I received a break when the newly hired Policy & Program Coordinator in the Centre for Students with Disabilities at my Alma Mater, with whom I had done a few disability awareness presentations, arranged with the Student Employment Centre to establish an accessible computer workstation to provide students with disabilities with access to employment information, resources and opportunities. The workstation, eventually named the BEA Station – Better Employment Access, needed a user manual and some promotional materials. The contract was mine if I wanted it.

This opportunity was ideal for me! It meant spending several days on campus, which was like going home again, to learn the specialized software for individuals with visual impairments. My eyes are one of my few body parts that work perfectly, so using the screen magnification and screen reader programs was a real eye-opener for me. I found it time-consuming, confusing, disorienting, and generally frustrating. It made me grateful and appreciative of my perfect vision.

Working at home, at my own pace and on my schedule, I researched and wrote the manual. I used email to connect with the Project Coordinator on a regular basis and whenever I had questions. It worked well. And the best part was that I submitted my hours and then received a cheque in the mail. *Real* money! It felt great.

As that project was wrapping up, I learned about a joint project between the Centre for Students with Disabilities and the Alumni Relations Office to make the current Career Mentor Program accessible to students and alumni with disabilities. This was an actual part-time job for one year; however, because of funding stipulations, it had to be posted, and the regular application and interview process was necessary. I began writing another cover letter, but this one had to be extremely good, without sounding desperate, because I *really* wanted this job.

The interview was with a panel of three people: the Alumni Relations Office's Executive Director, the Centre for Students with Disabilities' Policy & Program Coordinator, and the Neil Squire Foundation's Regional Manager, who was involved mainly to lend his expertise on accommodating candidates with disabilities in the interview process. While it was a bit of a relief that I knew people on the panel, if I failed in the interview, two of my colleagues would also know it. No pressure!

Realizing some candidates had stronger written communication skills than verbal ones, the interviewers gave a list of some questions ahead of time that we could respond to either in writing or verbally during the interview. These questions were in addition to questions asked verbally during the interview. This accommodation benefited me greatly as I could respond in greater detail in writing. It allowed for more of me to shine through, and it was a simple accommodation that didn't cost the employer anything.

Of all the jobs I had pursued, I felt most passionate about this one. I intensely understood the importance of establishing mentors for students with disabilities, something l would have liked at various points in my life.

My passion must have been obvious during the interview because I was offered the job! I was so excited! I felt like I could really add something to the Program. And, it also meant that I would no longer need social assistance, which I had been receiving since turning eighteen. Except for subsidized housing in that old folks' home, I would be flying on my own!

The first day or two of work were tense. The staff was trying so hard, perhaps even too hard, to do the *right* thing without being quite sure what was the *right* thing. At the end of my first day, my legs were sore from being so tight because everyone else was on edge. The following week, I sent around a memo, introducing myself and giving a few tips on how to deal with *Glenda-ish*. That broke the ice and helped everyone feel a bit more comfortable around me, allowing all of us to relax and do our jobs. Throughout the year, I did mini workshops at staff meetings to help increase disability awareness and comfort levels when interacting with people with disabilities.

As Project Coordinator, I worked closely with the Program Coordinator, Christopher, who I called Topher because it was much shorter for *Glenda-ish* to spit out. The Career Mentor Program was not a mentoring program in the typical sense. It was very focused on career exploration. Students usually met with a particular mentor only once, although they could meet with several mentors if they wished. Meetings generally took the form of informational interviews, where the student would ask about the mentor's job and duties, the education necessary, and career advancement possibilities.

My job was to make this program accessible and inclusive to people with disabilities. It was decided not to have two parallel programs, one for those with disabilities and one for those without, but to have one fully integrated program

Once I had *recruited* a fair number of mentors with disabilities, Topher and I organized a "Meet Your Mentor" lunch. With the lure of free pizza, which always seemed to bring out the students, we invited a panel of mentors with disabilities to share their stories with students with disabilities. Although we were working towards a fully integrated program, we felt that an event specifically for students with disabilities would make the students feel more comfortable in asking disability-related questions pertaining to employment so that they might begin exploring career options and opportunities.

The event went fairly well, considering it was our first one of that nature. While standing back and watching the mentors and students talk, Topher leaned on something as we chatted. He had a shock of a lifetime when he realized he was leaning on an *empty* wheelchair. His reaction was priceless! He then suggested the slogan for our next lunch should be "Come to a mentor lunch and be healed!" We had a good laugh. I then explained that some people who use wheelchairs and scooters are able to walk short distances, and thus, leave their wheelchairs behind while they mingle about the room. Even the Program Coordinator learned something that day.

Although I knew from day one that funding for my position was for only one year, I was sad that further funding was not found so that my position could continue. I had enjoyed my year, giving everything I had to make the project a success, and I still had ideas to continue growing the entire program. However, it was not meant to be.

The staff had a going-away potluck lunch, complete with cake and gifts from the campus bookstore. And, much to my utter surprise, Robin managed to pull off a home-warming/bridal shower in the boardroom. It was fantastic, and I appreciated all of the gifts, too. I was thankful for such a great year.

Then it was time to start the next chapter of my life. I had a life to build with Darrell, and the first order of business was to plan and organize the wedding for August.

ON A SEAT BUILT FOR TWO

In April, a two-bedroom "wheelchair-accessible" unit became available in his housing co-op. Although I wasn't overly keen about living together beforehand, we grabbed it, knowing such places were rare and that we may not find another one.

Dad came down for the weekend to move my belongings and then to begin moving Darrell's possessions across the complex. Darrell's parents were also down for the better part of the week to help us.

Sometime mid-week, Darrell's case manager from Long-Term Care came to reassess our need for homemaker services, as if moving in together had miraculously changed our need for service. She determined that we only needed basic housecleaning and laundry, not personal care. Big surprise! Then, amidst the unpacked boxes and unorganized clutter, she insisted on inspecting our home. She had to know the environment to which she would be sending homemakers and to check for safety issues. She was concerned about our shower arrangement.

The previous tenant had an attendant, and thus, had installed a roll-in shower. We simply put my shower bench against one wall, tied two large, grey cement bricks to the bench to anchor it down so it wouldn't tip over, and the maintenance guy installed a grab bar. Theoretically, we would park our chairs beside the bench, move ourselves onto the bench, pull the curtain, and....voila! Easy. But, because there were still boxes and parents everywhere, we had yet to put it to the test.

This case manager did not feel it was safe. Apparently, we weren't capable of deciding for ourselves whether it was safe or not, even though we knew our capabilities the best. I have bounced my head off cement floors enough times; I definitely would not put myself at risk needlessly.

This brilliant lady suggested sending in someone to be there when we showered. Now, I had only gained the privacy while showering a couple of years previously, and I wasn't about to give it up. To clarify her suggestion, I asked, "You are going to send someone in every day to watch us shower?" "Every day?" she asked, somewhat surprised by the frequency. I felt like asking, "Well, how often do you shower?" Besides, I didn't know if the hot water tank was big enough for two consecutive showers. She soon discarded that idea.

Then she suggested sending in an OT to assess the situation and offer any suitable suggestions. Now remember that I am not fond of OTs because I have yet to meet one who actually made sense. And, by this point I was rather prickly because she had dismissed my case manager's strong recommendation that I retain my homemaker. I finally had one that actually worked hard and understood written English, which was key for me since I often typed notes to communicate with my homemaker. For some bureaucratic reasons, it was not possible to keep Connie. However, I conceded to having an OT check out our shower. After all, Darrell and I wouldn't be bound to use any of the OT's recommendations; we would still have final say in what worked best for us for showering.

A month later, the OT visited. No, we didn't wait for a shower until then! We all traipsed into the bathroom. I felt like we should start charging admission! Her initial response to our arrangement was, "Don't know why I'm here. Looks like you have solved your own problem." Of course! Besides, I didn't recall having a problem! Her only suggestion was that suction-cup feet on the legs might hold the bench a bit firmer. She said she would get some. We are still waiting!

Back in the living room, she flipped through a few catalogs to see what other options existed. "Here's another option," she said as she passed the catalog over to us. Basically, it was a shelf that fastened to the wall. I took one look and, in my *Glenda-ish*, blurted out, "It won't hold two people!" Gasping in utter shock, she exclaimed, "Oh! I hadn't thought of that! You make me blush!" Flustered, she gathered up her things, saying, "I see I'm not needed here." She quickly departed, never to be heard from again.

Wedding Jitters

Driving along the highway and seeing the sun streaming through a cloud, I feel God. Walking through a forest with the sun filtering through the leaves, I feel God. Hearing the birds sing and seeing the flowers in bloom, I feel the presence of God. These are the reasons why I wanted my wedding, our wedding, outside in the spectacular beauty created by God Himself.

It wasn't that I didn't want a church wedding. It was simply that I wanted to be married where I felt closest to God. I knew that, for the most part, church aisles were not wide enough to accommodate two wheelchairs side-by-side, and I did not want to physically separate from my husband so soon after being wed. Heading down the aisle as a married couple only takes a brief moment, and then, once outside, Darrell and I could have rejoined. However, there are so many times in daily life that we must separate: going along the sidewalk, one is generally behind; on the bus, we are separated by the aisle; on the Skytrain, we sit at opposite ends of the car if we manage to get on the same car; and if we take a cab somewhere, we must take two because one cab can't take two wheelchairs. I did not want our wedding day to be like every other day.

A few people were disappointed that we didn't have a church wedding, which added to the stress of planning the day. Mom offered some advice by saying, "It is your wedding; do what feels right to you. I didn't raise you to fly

I'll Do It Myself

like an eagle only to have your wings clipped on your wedding day."

In the end, Darrell and I chose the Rose Garden atop Burnaby Mountain, overlooking Burrard Inlet. As I was working at SFU (also on Burnaby Mountain) at the time, colleagues drove me over one lunch hour to have a look, and then Darrell's parents drove us both up the next time they were in town. As soon as Darrell saw it, he agreed it was the place.

The actual day was beautiful. The roses were in full bloom. There wasn't a cloud in the sky. Many people asked me what we would do if it rained. I simply said, with definite certainty, "It won't rain on my wedding day." They were amazed at my confidence. The day was perfect, definitely one created by God.

The planning of the event was a little tricky. My Matron of Honour was in Hong Kong, and my bridesmaid was in Sydney on Vancouver Island (off the south coast of British Columbia). To add to the mayhem, both were named Karen. One Karen was my friend from Brownies; the other Karen was a childhood friend. Darrell's best man Tony lived in Nelson, in the southeastern corner of the province. And the usher/emcee, Darrell's brother Todd, and the ring bearer, our nephew Courtland, were in Crossett, Arkansas, in the United States. Talk about a spread out wedding party! Emails were flying around the world. The neat thing is that the Karens saved every email, printed them out, and presented them to me in a binder at the reception. I'll always treasure it.

Planning the wedding via email reminded me of a Communications project I had to do in university. Due to some accessibility issues late in the game, I had to change from a Publishing minor, which would be useful as I write this book, to a Communications minor. Unfortunately, it meant going back to take another first year Communications course in which we had a group project of planning and holding a dinner party with this group of people we didn't even know. Because of me and my *Glenda-ish*, our group was the first group to rely solely on email for communication in planning the party. Since then, I've used email to coordinate several groups, and I've laughed about that darn project each time. I never thought that lesson would be useful!

Keeping with tradition, I spent my last night of *singlehood* apart from Darrell. I spent the night at a motel suite down the street with my Mom and three brothers, a couple of significant others and one baby. Auntie Fern had a room a few doors down. It was great to have everyone together for that night. I truly appreciated that all three brothers were able to be there for my wedding day. It meant a lot to me.

We spent that night in the kitchen, preparing the food for the reception. Watching all three brothers peel pounds and pounds of potatoes for the potato salad, and cut and slice vegetables was amazing. It took their sister getting married for that to happen!

The next morning was a bit chaotic. With one bathroom for seven of us, it was like old times! Once we had the food prepared, the hair curled, the makeup applied, and the dress done up, it was time for even more pictures outside. Mom helped me into the car and organized my dressed. Suddenly I burst into unexplainable tears. A wave of mixed emotions overcame me. People kept taking pictures. I felt like Princess Di, with the paparazzi snapping pictures from every possible angle.

I'll Do It Myself

Karen's brother Kent was talked into being chauffer for the day. With signs "Honk for Glenda" and "Last Chance for Romance" on the car, he honked the horn the entire way up the mountain. Actually, it was kind of exciting! Mom followed with my scooter in her pickup and my brothers in their respective cars.

Across town at his sister's place, Dad was also experiencing chaos. Having left his dress shoes at home, he went out that morning to buy shoes, leaving clear instructions that everyone be ready for the wedding by the time he returned. As the story goes, no one was home when he returned. Instead, they had gone out for coffee without getting ready first. Dad, who usually doesn't get outwardly mad, was furious. He envisioned missing the chance to walk his only daughter down the aisle, being replaced by one of my brothers. Thankfully, everyone arrived at the Rose Garden safely and in time, and the ceremony proceeded as planned.

My gown was created by Mom, with love sewn into every stitch. Since I would be in my scooter, having a train was not possible. Mom came up with the brilliant idea to have an extremely long veil that flowed down from my red head to the ground, extending about six feet from my chair, about ten or twelve feet in length. She hand stitched countless seed pearls on to the veil for a special touch.

As there was a slight breeze, the Karens held my veil as if it was a train to keep it from blowing around. With the instrumental version of Bryan Adam's "(Everything I Do) I Do It for You" playing in the background, the bridal party of four proceeded down the aisle, a rose arbour laden in full blossoms that was absolutely beautiful. I felt like a princess that day.

With our families and friends gathered around us, Darrell and I exchanged vows that we had written ourselves. We purposefully omitted the traditional "promising to obey," which was too archaic for me. We did vow, in part, to encourage one another, to communicate openly and honestly, and to accept the other, now and in the future, while still remaining true to ourselves.

Soon after being pronounced husband and wife by the Marriage Commissioner, the Karens tied heart-shaped "Just Married" signs to the backs of our wheelchairs, along with strings of pop cans that dragged on the ground behind us.

The reception was held in the small hall in our housing co-op. Because it was a sunny, beautiful day as I had planned, the tables were set up on the large patio, giving us a little more room. Operating on a shoestring budget, the tables were covered in newsprint, with crayons placed on each table to entertain young and old alike! Paper and pens were also on each table for adults to share their pearls of wisdom on a successful marriage. We still have these treasures. Many people commented on how our wedding was so relaxed and enjoyable. I'm not sure if every bride hears that or if our wedding was actually something different.

Dad built a wooden arch, wide enough for two wheelchairs, under which Darrell and I sat while handing out pieces of wedding cake to our guests. The three-layer wedding cake was Mom's grandpa's fruitcake recipe from his bake shop, a recipe Mom had used over the years for her delicious Christmas cake.

With a fair amount of food left over, more than could fit in our small freezer, Mom and Kevin made a late night delivery to a local homeless shelter. Sharing our happy day with those who were less fortunate than us meant a lot to me and made the day even more memorable.

One of my fondest memories is of my bridesmaid Karen teaching my Grandma – with facial lines of experience, wisdom and beauty, and crinkly gray hair, as one brother had once described it – the Macarena Dance. Hesitant and uncertain at first, she soon caught on. Karen created a special moment that I will cherish for the rest of my days.

As the evening came to a close, our families and friends sent us off into the married world. To be environmentally friendly, my bridesmaid Karen and her two young daughters, Kimberly and Ashley, made bundles of bird seed, rather than rice, to throw at us. Darrell and I had bird seed everywhere: down our clothes, in our mouths, and everywhere!

We were now married, and we will spend the rest of our lives learning and discovering what that actually meant, in bad times and in good.

The Eagle Takes Flight

Newly married, our next task was to find employment as both of our Employment Insurance claims were running out. We both had been unemployed for several months with no prospects. We both had no doubt that our disabilities had something to do with our unemployment status; proving that was another story. After all, that would have meant discrimination, which is illegal.

After much thought and without any opportunities presenting themselves, I decided to take the plunge and start my own business. I had been considering it for a few years, and now seemed the perfect time to do it. Being self-employed, I could work from home, which would save the hassle of a commute, and I could work flexible hours as long as the work was done on time. It seemed like a sensible way to *accommodate my disability*.

I began researching self-employment programs. I knew of one specifically for people with disabilities, but that didn't appeal to me. I didn't want a watered down program, which is why I was hesitant of a program for only people with disabilities. In my mind, that was like going back to Special Ed class, which I had left behind long ago. I wanted to do this right.

I chose the Self Employment Program through Douglas College, attended the information session in mid-September and picked up the application, which was a sixteen-page form due in ten days. Because I didn't have the form in electronic format, I first had to recreate it on my computer so that I could then begin filling it out. The application was essentially a rough business plan – in ten days! Our honeymoon was over!

Once I completed and submitted the intensive application form, I was called for the next step in the application process. Armed with my handy alphabet card, I met with an assigned business advisor to discuss my business idea. October 7th I received the news that I had been accepted into the program! I soon realized the application was the easy part; now began the *real* work.

The day after receiving the news, I received an email from my business advisor with a long list of questions about my disability and how to best accommodate me in the classroom. Liberally copied (and slightly edited) from the email message, which I have saved all these years for this very purpose, the questions included the following:

1. Do you have any personal needs that we should be aware of? I'm thinking of help to and from the bus, washrooms, and assistance to eat – if class is long you may wish to eat lunch at the cafeteria, etc.

2. Do you require any adaptive equipment to participate in our program? I haven't any idea what that might be. It seemed to me that you were very organized and self-contained in the times we met. However, with your experience at SFU you probably know exactly what you need for the classroom setting. Please identify anything that we might provide.

3. Which brings to mind another somewhat obvious question...Is there anything that we need to know about you or your condition that may assist us in helping you learn? I didn't notice it, but someone asked me if you also had difficulty hearing – if so, tell us how we can help you.

4. Many of our classes are highly participative. We have small group discussions and people talk with each other about their business plans. Sometimes these are the times of greatest learning for participants. How would this work for you? We, of course, want YOU to be able to tell others about your business ideas, and to hear about your thoughts on the matters being discussed. Any suggestions for our facilitators?

And the list continued. However, I do give my business advisor and the rest of the staff credit for asking the questions. It is better for people to bluntly ask questions than to bumble along, operating on the basis of false assumptions and misconceptions about my disability. Although, I did sense the questions were put forth to alleviate the staff's potential fears of the *unknown* as much as they were to best accommodate me. Taking a deep breath, I began typing responses to my business advisor's questions, beginning with the word "RELAX!" I chuckled at some of the questions; once again, my hearing and cognitive abilities were questioned because of my physical disability. I have no doubt my business advisor met with the college's Disabled Student Services Coordinator, who planted some of these questions and concerns in her mind. Once again, I would have to prove my capabilities to another group of adults. All I wanted to do was to learn how to run my own business!

Ironically, part of my business idea was disability awareness training. During the months I was in the program, I was also indirectly *training* the staff and fellow students – one of those free services self-employed people provide in order to generate new business.

Classes were held way out at the Coquitlam campus rather than the New Westminster one, which would have been fairly simple to get to by Skytrain. Travelling to Coquitlam made for rather early mornings as I was up between 4:00am and 4:30am to be out of the house by 6:30am at the latest. Because I need nearly two hours to get ready in the morning, I had learned at university to avoid registering for 8:30 classes whenever possible! And that was when I was living on campus, a few minutes from class! I now faced a solid hour or more bus ride (with a transfer), leaving enough time for any bus mishaps, like the wheelchair lift not working and needing to wait for the next bus (or two). I would arrive at the college around 8:00, in time for a bathroom break before class at 8:30am. But, compared to a few years earlier when I was stuck atop Burnaby Mountain for weeks at a time, it was an improvement. At least I *could* get out to Coquitlam by myself. It simply made for awfully early mornings!

I was home by mid-afternoon, and Darrell would have an early supper nearly ready. I then stretched out on the couch for a couple hours to *watch* the news – with my eyes closed! It was then time to do that dreaded h-word – homework (like I hadn't done enough in my lifetime!). Around midnight, exhausted and bleary-eyed, I would fall into bed briefly before beginning the process over again.

Thankfully, I had to keep that schedule only during the Business Plan Development phase of the program, in which I researched and wrote a 36-page business plan in three weeks. My poor left thumb was flying to keep up with the brutal pace! The Business Training phase, in which we learned how to operate and market our business, was at a more manageable pace. Also, by then my business advisor and the program manager had found some funding through the Opportunity Fund, a Canadian government program to assist people with disabilities in obtaining employment or self-employment, to pay for a wheelchair taxi, which saved me some travel time and was much appreciated.

My business idea stemmed from an interest sparked a few years earlier. While taking the pre-employment program at the Neil Squire Foundation, the instructors were soon scrambling to keep me busy and suitably challenged. One day the computer instructor introduced me to basic HTML for designing websites. I gobbled it up! I soon realized that, although I grew up in silence, I now had a way to communicate with the world. That realization was so exciting, so liberating!

I continued learning HTML on my own and came across the term web accessibility. Like the real world, the internet also presented barriers to people with disabilities if particular guidelines weren't followed. As I did more reading and learning, I understood that, although using the internet didn't pose insurmountable barriers for me, people with other kinds of disabilities would have problems using it.

These problems existed because web developers and decision-makers were not aware of the need for making websites accessible. To make sure other people with disabilities had the same freedom and opportunities provided to me by the internet, I wanted to assist organizations with making their websites accessible to everyone, regardless of an individual's abilities or the technology used. By making their websites accessible, businesses would increase the number of people capable of accessing their sites and, in turn, increase their customer base, which translates into increased profits. Their corporate image would improve because no group, including their own employees with disabilities, would be excluded from using the website.

My business plan also included adding disability awareness training and potentially Braille printing (embossing) services in the future. My mission was to increase awareness and accessibility of communication so that people with disabilities may fully participate in all facets of society. My guiding principle was something I dubbed the AAA Principle: *accessibility* also involves *awareness* and *acceptance* of people with disabilities – all disabilities.

I then needed a suitable business name, which took more thought than I realized it would. I was sitting in our rather overstuffed dining room/living room with my *office* nestled at the end, in front of the large window. Over our faux fireplace hung a beautifully cross-stitched picture of an eagle with wings spread, a wedding gift from Auntie Fern's then partner's father. It hit me – Eagle Communications. The eagle represented strength, grace, independence and power to me. Also, as I was growing up, Mom had often said she tried to give me eagle wings so that I could fly. The "Communications" portion of the name was general enough to allow my business to grow, as long as it was related to some aspect of communications. Eventually Eagle Communications became Soaring Eagle Communications, giving a stronger image of strength, independence and grace.

The Business Training phase of the program ended shortly before Christmas. We then had support from our business advisors for another nine months as we worked to launch our businesses. In March, I landed my first paying project with a local dot com company. My challenge was to develop guidelines for choosing website colour schemes that would be readable by people who were colour blind. Essentially, I was to write a report on a topic I knew absolutely nothing about, as I had done for seven years in university. *Fake it till you make it* became my new mantra. But this time, I would be paid for it!

As I began digging into the issue, I discovered that little research had been done on it at that time. After asking questions via email of various people in the field, I developed guidelines for choosing colour schemes for people with colour blindness. The next project was to actually choose several colour schemes, which were then implemented on the Government of British Columbia's website. That was quite a "heady" experience to visit the provincial government's site and see my colour choices being used. I had accomplished something and had made a difference for those people who have trouble distinguishing different colours, which is approximately eight percent of males and one percent of females, according to my research.

With those two small projects under my belt, I thought I was on a roll. But I soon realized it was beginner's luck. Having a new business with relatively few contacts, being non-verbal, and working in a field about which most people had no knowledge didn't make a great combination for instant business success. As with any business, particularly with a fledgling business like mine, networking is crucial. I did attend a few networking events sponsored by the Self-Employment Program, but I found they weren't highly effective without verbal communication. I even tried printing my business information on postcard-sized cards and handing them to people who stopped to talk, but the cards had very limited success.

I was intimidated to wheel into a room of people standing and milling about because my eye level was their fly level, so making eye contact was difficult. Most people walk into a room and notice how many people are wearing glasses; I wheel in and notice how many flies are undone – a surprising number! With my current scooter I am at breast height. It's not exactly a thrilling perspective for me, but I am moving on up in the world!

The other problem was my actual business. *What is web accessibility?* People understand the need for making buildings accessible, but websites? *Isn't using the internet as simple as point and click? What do you mean blind people can use computers? How do they see the screen or type? Text-to-speech screen readers? Refreshable Braille displays?* People would get a glazed look on their faces, say "Oh, that's interesting," and then move on to the next entrepreneur to practice their own thirty-second business spiel. Forget the idea of meeting someone for coffee or lunch to discuss potential opportunities for forming strategic alliances or joint ventures! And, until we got a cable internet connection at home, my business phone line was only used for internet connection. I was terrified to answer that phone. A heavy-breathing, inaudible voice answering the phone would likely kill any potential business opportunity!

But, in typical, stubborn-headed Glenda-fashion, I persevered. The Eagle struggled to find its wings. I landed a few small projects through the remainder of the year; some dealt with web accessibility, some did not. And I did quite a bit of increasing awareness and indirectly educating people around the issue of web accessibility and the need for developing accessible websites.

In April, Darrell decided to also apply to the Self Employment Program as a means of creating work for himself. No other employment opportunities had presented themselves, but it wasn't for a lack of trying on his part. He began the brutal Business Plan Development process, but this time we knew what to expect since I could share my own experiences. Also, the Opportunity Fund was accessed almost immediately this time, saving Darrell the long commutes each day.

I realized that, even though we both have cerebral palsy, we are treated so differently. When I was going through the first phase, the other participants seldom interacted with me, which was nothing new for me. But, once I had completed my business plan and had been approved by the Local Review Committee, the litmus test for getting into the second phase of the program, they began interacting and conversing with me. Even one of the advisors admitted that the facilitators weren't sure I was *understanding it* until they read my business plan. Once again I had to prove myself and my abilities to be taken seriously.

Yet, with Darrell, fellow classmates were talking and joking with him on the first day of class before he had written a single sentence. I have no doubt that his clear speech is the major reason for the difference in how people interact with us. It still baffles me how or why people assume that unclear speech means cognitive deficiencies. And, because *they* can't understand me, why do they assume I am the one with the cognitive impairment or hearing impairment?

Somewhere along the way, as we were both struggling to get our businesses going, we found ourselves caught in limbo between federal and provincial programs. Because two levels of governments were involved and the situation was complex, no one could *really* guide us through the maze of red tape. No one had ever taken a federally funded self employment program while on provincial social assistance and classified as "Disability Level II"; in fact, according to our social worker, this was something I was not even allowed to do "according the legislation". I was waiting for the RCMP to arrest me for trying to start my own business.

Darrell and I were extremely stressed, as if being newlyweds and trying to start two businesses from one home wasn't difficult enough! We had to rely on each other because no one else completely understood our predicament. When one was down, the other would be up. Thank goodness we were never both down at the same time! I'm not sure what would have happened. It sure felt like the Ministry was trying to keep us oppressed, caught in the social assistance system. Never once did anyone from the Ministry say, "It's great that you're starting your own business. How may we help you be a success?" They kept putting barriers in front of us, saying we couldn't do it.

I was not raised to have this attitude, and it went against everything in which I believed. Why wouldn't they support me if I wanted to try being self-employed? To me, running my own business from home was a potentially viable alternative to employers not eager to hire me, and it meant I could work on my own schedule when my energy was high. With my limited energy due to my physical disability, I knew I couldn't physically handle a full-time job. Self-employment made sense to me. I was trying to get off social assistance, yet they would not help me to accomplish that goal.

A paralegal from Legal Aid gave us some assistance, but even she didn't fully understand the complexities of the situation. I had to point out many of the twists and turns to her. We went to tribunal and won, and the Ministry subsequently appealed and lost. But these were empty victories for us because they resulted in nothing. The Ministry didn't deliver what they were suppose to as laid out in the decision, and by then we were too worn out to fight any more without serious help behind us. Shortly afterward, Darrell landed a part-time job, which eventually became full-time, at the Neil Squire Foundation. We welcomed the steady income and tried to simply move forward and put that whole mess behind us.

The following spring, I became the BC Coordinator for WORKink, an online employment resource centre for people with disabilities; an initiative of the Canadian Council on Rehabilitation and Work. The position didn't exactly involve web accessibility, but it was something I *could* do and something that could be, for the most part, done from home. This was my first taste of working with a virtual team. Our monthly meetings were held using an online text chat room. We typed our thoughts, rather than speaking them. This approach accommodated me with my speech impairment, the two members with hearing impairments, and the one with a sight impairment whose screen reader was compatible with the text chat software. It was quite an effective way to accommodate our various disabilities. Unfortunately, as is typical with many programs for people with disabilities, my position was dependent upon funding that disappeared after a year. I learned that a signed contract doesn't always mean a job. That steady income was gone.

From there, I landed occasional government contracts, which were quite challenging and fairly lucrative. In fact, we were able to save enough for a down payment to buy our own home, a condo in Surrey, not far from where I had started school many years ago. Most of the projects stemmed from budgets that needed to be spent by fiscal year-end, so they were left until the last minute. Poor planning by the client meant many late nights and all-nighters on my part! But, thanks to my supportive husband who picks up the cooking duties, calms me when I panic, and then gives me the space and time to do what I need to do, I have never missed a deadline.

As I write this, I sense the Eagle is about to change directions. Although I have done some interesting work and have become somewhat known in the web accessibility field, I don't think I have yet hit my full potential. Because the work has been fairly sporadic, I feel it is time to explore other opportunities. The future is mine. I simply need to take the knowledge and experience gained from eight years of self-employment, combine that with the latest technologies and new opportunities, and then the Eagle will spread its wings, catch an updraft and truly soar to heights that are yet unimaginable!

From the Heart

Toxic black mould had spread throughout the housing complex and was causing health concerns for Darrell and me, particularly with my weakened lung capacity. As a satisfactory remedy was not imminent, our only option was to move. We began exploring other housing co-operatives; but the waiting lists were long, and some places were less desirable than ours. The next step was to seriously consider buying our own home. Financially, it made more sense to put money into a mortgage and build equity rather than to pay rent and be guaranteed a roof over our heads for only another month. We applied for a mortgage through one bank and were told we qualified on the condition that we had a co-signer, which we did not consider an acceptable solution. We had no doubt that our wheelchairs played a role in the bank's decision. We decided to try again in one year.

In the spring of 2001, we applied again for a mortgage; this time we applied through a mortgage broker. We were approved! We went home-hunting and, after viewing several places, found a spacious, two-bedroom condominium that I instantly knew was our new home. The unit on the top floor of a three-storey building was airy and bright with its southwest-facing windows, and nearly 1400 square feet was enough space for Darrell's two wheelchairs and my two scooters. The only required adaptation was installing two grab bars in the en suite bathroom.

After living in our new home for a few months, we realized that the thick carpet was too hard on Darrell's shoulders when wheeling his manual chair; and it burned out the motor on my little Amigo scooter. The carpet was replaced with parquet hardwood flooring, which Dad installed over the next several months.

One day, I was down on my hands and knees, trying to help Dad put rollers under the freezer to move it out of the dining room. Suddenly, I was out of breath and my heart was racing. This had happened once a few weeks earlier when trying to lift a bag of used clothes into a donation bin.

I had recently seen Oprah's show on the prevalence of, yet often misdiagnosed, heart disease among women, so I did not argue this time when Darrell offered to make a doctor's appointment. I kept thinking of my friend Karen. I was scared.

Karen was a few years older than I and had severe athetoid cp. She was completely dependent on others for all her needs. Her feet and hands were usually strapped down to prevent them from flying about. Yet, she always had a big smile.

In her early twenties, she began developing scoliosis, a curvature in her back. It became so bad that she couldn't digest her food properly, so she would end up throwing up when put to bed. Eventually the surgeon inserted a Harrington rod to straighten her spine.

Four days before my high school Grad Banquet and Dance, as we were getting ready for school, the phone rang, which was a very rare occurrence that early in the morning. It was Karen's mom. Karen had pulled through the surgery quite nicely, and she was even beginning to sit up in the hospital bed. But early that morning she went into cardiac arrest. She did not survive.

I was very upset, but our family didn't stop for death, for some unknown reason. Off to school I went. I told only one friend about Karen. After that morning, Karen wasn't spoken of much again. Her parents, my second mom, were never heard from again, and there was no mention of a funeral or a memorial service. But I didn't forget her. I know she is one of my guardian angels.

I was surprised that someone so young could die from a heart attack, and that thought has always stayed with me. Thus, between Karen's story, Oprah's show and my racing heart, I was willing to go to the doctor. He listened to my heart and then sent me for a blood test and an EKG, which was an adventure with athetoid cp. When I saw the screen, I thought I definitely had a problem. Then after several long minutes, the lab technician mentioned that the machine picks up every little muscle movement; ignore all those extra spikes. She told me to relax, which is easier said than done!

In the end, the test results confirmed the doctor's hunch: I had a healthy heart, but it was unfit. Then he said something that a medical professional had never before said to me. Darrell and I could expect to live a normal life span if we took care of ourselves from that point forward. He recommended twenty minutes of cardio-vascular exercise three times each week.

During my years at SFU, I came across a book on cp that said the life expectancy was thirty years. Although, rationally, I knew that was an old statistic and not necessarily true, I felt like I was living on borrowed time. Karen's story and others simply reconfirmed that feeling.

After the doctor's visit, the reason for Karen's death suddenly became clearer, at least in my own mind. Learning about anorexia and bulimia in my Psychology courses, I had rationalized that her constant throwing up and her thinness due to her cp probably had a similar effect on her heart as would an actual eating disorder. This condition combined with her inability to be physically active did not allow her heart to survive the surgical assault on her body.

Exercise is one of those things you "should do" amongst all of the other "should do's", but I never truly appreciated the importance of exercise. For people with disabilities, exercise is generally framed as therapy or rehabilitation. Boring! I have rarely seen exercise for people with disabilities framed in terms of fitness or general well-being.

Dr. Golin's words gave me a new perspective on life. I can take an active role in preventing heart disease, and I can plan on living a long, fulfilling life.

Baby, Baby, Baby

My friend recently told me that she is pregnant with her fourth child. Earlier that day, she had her first ultrasound, and she saw the baby's heartbeat. She cried. I told her that I was happy for her. I cried.

Why does each subsequent pending birth announcement from family and friends cut deeper and deeper into my soul, into my being? I will never know the miracle and wonder of a life beginning within me: the movement, the growth, the discomfort. I will never know the awesome feeling of bringing a new being into the world or the overwhelming responsibility of having a little person completely and utterly dependent upon me.

I will never hear the patter of little feet coming down the hall in the morning. I will never kiss boo boos and scare away terrifying monsters. I will never stay up all night making angel wings or dinosaur tails. I will never have handprints on my fridge or spilled juice on the couch. I will never wait up on the first date. I will never cry buckets as my little miracle goes off into the world. And, I will never know the heartbreak, disappointment and grief if life doesn't go as I dreamed, hoped and prayed for this miracle.

I will never know because I will never give life to a little miracle. I will never be pregnant. Not by choice. It is how things are for Darrell and me. A few relatives have even told me not to get pregnant, not knowing that Darrell cannot make a child. They are unaware of how much it hurts to hear that advice from people who love us. And, with my cp, I'm not sure that I could even carry a baby full-term. I don't know how being pregnant would affect my cp or how my cp would affect the baby.

I don't know how the two of us would care for a baby, including the diaper changing, the bathing, the feeding, the lifting, the chasing – I'm not sure how we would manage.

But that isn't to say Darrell and I wouldn't love to have our own child. We would. We have often talked about how we would be good parents. I tease Darrell that he would spoil them because he is such a softie. He says, according to his grandma, there is no such thing as spoiling, just "love lots". We definitely would *love lots*.

We have often cried together as we watch news stories of horrific tragedies that have befallen children, oftentimes at the hand of a parent, relative or friend that should have done everything humanly possible to protect, care for and love them. It seems so unfair that we can't have children, yet others don't realize and appreciate the precious gift they have when they have a child.

This is probably one of the most difficult things that both Darrell and I, both as a couple and as individuals, have had to deal with related to our cerebral palsy. For the most part, I have lived a fairly *normal* life and have done many of the things my friends and peers have done. This one thing makes me unable to fully share and connect with my girlfriends on that level. I don't have those experiences and feelings to share with them. Being childless can make for rather one-sided conversations at times.

I recall one time in particular being at my friend Barb's house during my first year at university; her brother, wife and baby were also there. Somehow I ended up sitting on the couch, holding Christina. She was between six and nine months old, a more responsive age beyond that *extremely fragile* stage when I'm afraid that I'm going to hurt them. Everyone else was busy around the house. Christina soon fell asleep in my arms, and I sat there, holding her.

I gazed out the living room window, thinking and wondering about my future. Something told me I would probably never have children, mainly because, at that time, I thought I would never get married. A feeling of sadness and emptiness came over me, a feeling that is still there today when I pay attention to it. Barb came by a while later to ask if I wanted her to take the baby so that I could move. I said, "No, I'm fine." I was thinking, *No, please don't take her. Please let me have this time with her.* I swallowed the lump in my throat and blinked away the tear that was about to escape down my cheek.

The condo Darrell and I bought is great for us – spacious, bright, accessible, and close to shopping and transit. The one drawback is that it's a "mature complex"; in other words, no children are allowed. Our four brothers and their families live elsewhere, so we perform our auntie and uncle duties across the miles for our eleven nieces and nephews: Courtland, Alie, Dameon, Trenton, Cheyenne, Nicole, Robin, Victoria, Madison, Sydney and Hannah. My brother Ian insisted that Hannah and I share the same middle name, Louise, and I was deeply touched that he felt so strongly about it.

Regrettably, Darrell and I don't even have surrogate children around to *love lots*. But, on those occasions when we do see them, we savour every moment of their boundless energy, their inquisitive *why* and *how* questions, their delight to sit on our laps as Darrell and I race each other along the sidewalk, and their desire to feel safe and to be heard by adults. These are memories Darrell and I will dearly cherish for the rest of our days.

UNENLIGHTENED SOULS

One day when Darrell and I were house hunting, his wheelchair died. He had to take a taxi home. Since our local taxis can only hold one wheelchair, I took the Skytrain home alone. I had done it a million times before. The train car was fairly empty, and I was sitting there, minding my own business. I guess my face was twitching a bit as it does with athetoid cp, because as one woman got off at her stop, she commented, "Pretty weird face you got there," as she purposefully made facial grimaces. Then she asked, "Are you retarded?" Instantly I was transported back to that day in Grade 4 or 5.

Mom taught at my elementary school, so she would pick me up from my classroom at the end of the day and carry me out to the van at the front of the school; the school wheelchair stayed at school. One day, Mom had to stop at the office on our way out. She sat me down on the floor in the hall next to the gym doors at the main entrance. She would be only a couple of minutes, and I wasn't in the way as people were leaving.

One boy, a year or two older than me, walked by and asked, "Are you retarded?" and then kept walking. I didn't know what to say, and if I had said anything, my speech would have added fuel to the fire and would have confirmed his assumption. I said nothing.

Once Mom put me into the van, I burst into tears. When I managed to stop crying enough to communicate what had happened, Mom was sympathetic. She attempted to make light of it like she usually does, suggesting that next time I reply with something like, "No, are you?" – as if I could get that out clearly enough for it to be effective.

The incident was soon brushed off and forgotten – on the outside; but it wasn't forgotten on the inside. That question hurt me to my core for a long, long time. Even though I knew I wasn't retarded, I realized that others did see me as something I'm not. Since that day, I've been trying hard to prove to others that I'm not retarded.

This time, on the Skytrain, I didn't dare look away or down; otherwise, she would have won. I maintained unwavering eye contact during the entire insult. She continued, "Are you retarded? What is your problem?" I responded firmly, "No. You," meaning *she* was my problem. But I doubt she understood my intended message. She finally departed and the Skytrain continued.

Behind my sunglasses fell an odd tear that escaped down my cheek. It seemed like a long ride home. I burst into tears as soon as I opened our front door. I guess my university degree, marriage and pending homeownership didn't prove anything. In the eyes of many people, I was still that kid sitting on the floor in the school hallway.

Another unenlightened soul is permanently etched in my memory. Mom and I had stopped at Safeway to buy a few things. I was in my small, red wheelchair; pushing it and a shopping cart was a tricky maneuver for Mom, but she managed. At the checkout, which had the old, curved-style counter with a separate pass-thru for the carts, my wheelchair would not fit through the curved aisle. Mom told the cashier that she would wheel me around all the checkouts to the other end of the counter and then pay for the groceries. An old man behind us in the line suggested that Mom simply push me through where the carts went.

Mom promptly responded, "She is not a sack of potatoes!" and wheeled me around. Again, I did not show how much that encounter hurt me until we were safely inside the van.

More recently, when Darrell and I finally met some of our neighbours in the condo, one neighbour mentioned that he had seen me from a distance at the shopping mall a few weeks previously. He was surprised that I was out shopping alone. He didn't think I could do that. What I found most annoying was that, before even meeting me and knowing me, he had made assumptions about me, my disability and my capabilities. And, he interacted with me based on those wrong assumptions and misconceptions until I could prove myself differently to him. I get weary having to enlighten every soul I encounter.

Sometimes I tend to retreat to the safety of our own home, where I am not insulted and prejudged and can simply be me. However, I must contend with the phone, which isn't always a friend to someone whose speech is difficult to understand. Because of my breathy voice, some telemarketers are concerned that I'm hurt or sick and are about ready to call 911 until I reassure them that I am truly fine. I don't mind them as much as the obnoxious ones who intrude upon the safety and refuge of my home by insulting me when they don't understand me, like a guy representing the Chamber of Commerce who called me a "fucking retard". Thank you for interrupting my peace and solitude for that.

I accept that when I go outside my front door, I am at risk of stares, comments and insults from complete strangers who, for the most part, do not know any better. Unfortunately, that is part of living life with a disability, and I try to ignore them outwardly. They still hurt me on the inside. For this reason, I value the safety and solitude of my four walls. It is when a stranger on the other end of the phone intrudes upon my private space and verbally attacks me that I really hurt, and the frustration builds.

Equally frustrating is when someone who hasn't been forewarned about my speech calls for Darrell, and the person won't talk to me because I am not understandable. I feel like a failure because I can't take a phone message for my husband. It can bring me down briefly, until I shake myself out of it.

Regrettably, a young girl received the brunt of the years of built-up frustration. She kept phoning mid-afternoon, no doubt calling a friend after school and misdialing the number, repeatedly. When she asked for her friend Sarah, I simply said "No" and hung up. But when she kept calling and asking for Sarah after repeated no's at an increasing volume, I got so frustrated that I banged the phone on the counter several times before hanging up. I confess that it did feel good in the moment. Afterwards I felt guilty, hoping I hadn't deafened the poor girl or caused a lifetime phone phobia. It was not one of my proudest moments. I was simply at my wit's end.

Healing Hands

As I began sensing the time was right to start writing this book, my left hand, my typing hand, started protesting. *I have been working since I was five, with no real appreciation. I think I'll force Glenda to stop for a while.* My fingers were tingling and going numb, and my wrist and knuckles were fairly painful. Simple things, such as picking up cans while grocery shopping, were becoming difficult. And using the computer, particularly the mouse, was causing pain.

I was scared; in fact, I was terrified. Writing, in whatever format, was my predominant means of income. If I could no longer type, how would I earn a living? I was only thirty-six and still had a career or two ahead of me. Flipping burgers, pumping gas or performing brain surgery were definitely not options for me. What was I going to do? I felt like God was playing a cruel joke on me, and I didn't know what to do.

I had been typing since age five; it was part of me. The typed word is my connection with and contribution to society. Without it I would have nothing of value to offer to society or, perhaps, nothing society would see as valuable. Without the typed word, I would be isolated from society, except for those few who understand or who take the time to learn *Glenda-ish*. Without the typed word, I have no means of expressing myself; I merely survive, with no tangible way of recording or marking my existence.

Since not typing was NOT an option, I had to find another method or two for typing and using a mouse. I returned to the Neil Squire Foundation, where they specialize in assistive technology (AT) to aid people with disabilities in using computers and where Darrell happened to work at that time. The AT Specialist, Patricia, and I began exploring possible solutions.

One solution was the Penny & Giles joystick, a very solid joystick with *grooves* that improve my control despite my jerky movements; it could work in place of the mouse and in conjunction with an onscreen keyboard. Unfortunately, it was too expensive to justify since I was not working. However, without it I would be in too much pain to work the next time a paying project presented itself. After several months, I conceded. Darrell placed the order, but only after he demonstrated how we could pay off the Visa bill by dipping into our wedding gift money. He was being a good husband, trying to do what was best for his wife long term, and I was giving him grief over a few hundred dollars. Life with me isn't always easy!

Patricia and I also experimented with Dragon Dictate, voice recognition software that we hoped would reliably recognize how I said each letter so that I could verbally spell the words. Training the software took me back to my speech therapy days, except this was high tech therapy, and I didn't need to lay on the floor with stinky toes in my face. The software recognized the first few letters that I trained. It was looking hopeful! But as I trained more letters, the software became more and more confused, and the recognition rate decreased significantly.

We then tried Dragon Dictate with EZ Keys, software that I had been using for a couple of years for word prediction and completion, which saved me a fair bit of typing. We discovered instantly that the two pieces of software were not compatible, as a siren alarm started blaring from the computer speakers. Obviously, that combination was not an effective solution! Next.

As one last experiment to make sure we hadn't left any stone unturned, I tried the Jouse, a device actually developed by the Foundation and mainly used by individuals with high-level spinal cord injuries with virtually no hand function. This device enables them to control the mouse with their mouth and to enter text via Morse code using the sip and puff method. The Jouse requires good head and breath control, neither of which I have. And, when I inadvertently pulled out the short, plastic straw, which I then could have easily swallowed, with my teeth, it was obvious that the Jouse was not an option for me.

With the current state of assistive technology, this left me with only my new joystick and potentially an onscreen keyboard as an alternative to typing. And this would have to suffice until my *cap* is invented. A cap that would read my thoughts and type them directly into the computer is something that I have dreamed about since I was ten years old. I am convinced that if I wore the cap at night, when most of my creative thoughts come to me, and then edited the text in the morning, I would accomplish so much more. I need to be patient for technology to catch up to my quirky needs. Regardless, I still think my left thumb will always feel the most natural.

Whenever a possible solution didn't work, it was somewhat disheartening; it meant my options were decreasing. During this journey, I also went the medical route to determine what was wrong physically. X-rays and blood tests ruled out arthritis, which was a relief!

Next was the EMG (electromyography) to test the functioning of nerves. With electrodes fastened from a computer to my wrist and arm, which the lab technician then zapped repeatedly, I felt like I was in Frankenstein's lab. I jumped higher with each subsequent shock. From my perspective, my nerve function was working quite well! I felt each shock, and each one DID hurt!

Results indicated mild carpel tunnel syndrome, which was no surprise; I suspected I had it. They also suspected tendonitis, and I wondered what torture test was needed to confirm that possibility. Before the actual test, the medical specialist asked me a series of questions on the functioning and degree of pain in my left hand. When he attempted to examine my right hand, which is either a tightly clenched fist or, when opened, a dropped wrist with fingers pointing every which way, he asked if I had ever tried Botox or if it had even been suggested before. He offered that Botox might reduce the tightness so that perhaps functioning could be increased.

Within five minutes he had made a judgment call about my quality of life. He didn't ask if I was happy with my level of functioning; he simply assumed I should have more. I can control my scooter, hold the reins, pull up my pants and hit pretty hard with that hand. What else do I need to do with my right hand? I doubted a Botox injection would enable me to cut my food or type with that hand, so what was the point? And, especially when the long-term effects of Botox were still unknown, I wasn't overly keen on becoming a human guinea pig when I had been fairly content with my hand up until that appointment. I began doubting myself, wondering if I should be expecting more from my right hand.

I appreciated that he offered a potential solution, as any good doctor should, but I felt like he was suggesting a solution before confirming the problem. I felt like he was treating the medical condition without dealing with the person. In my mind, it seemed like he was attempting to heal the wrong hand.

Around this time, I learned that I also have fairly severe osteoporosis. This was a bigger shock to me than to my family doctor because it's common knowledge in the medical profession that spending a lifetime in a wheelchair with minimal walking puts one at great risk of osteoporosis. This fact was not shared with me by any of the many doctors who I had seen in my lifetime, and I doubt it would have come up at that time either had I not asked about calcium supplements as a preventative measure since menopause probably wasn't too far away.

If I had known that I was at risk of developing osteoporosis because I wasn't physically active, I could have made some informed decisions in my younger years. I probably would have made a conscious effort to be more active. Perhaps I would have spent a little less time in my bedroom doing homework during my school years. Perhaps I would have aimed to have a more balanced life. But, without that information, I could not make that decision. I was mad at my current doctor as well as all the doctors through my lifetime for not having discussed this *with me* previously. I do remember one E.R. doctor, after examining a leg x-ray, mentioning that I had fine bones, like an astronaut. I thought that was interesting, but I didn't realize the significance of that comment or think to pursue it further. After all, I was the patient, not the doctor!

Once I was diagnosed in May 2003, I began researching osteoporosis to gain a better understanding of what was happening in my body, since my family doctor didn't bother explaining it to me. Perhaps he thought I wouldn't understand or that I had no interest in knowing how my body works, but he didn't ask if I was interested either. He simply prescribed Fosamax.

I learned that bone is continually regenerating itself. The bone cells' osteoclasts slough off old bone cells, and then osteoblasts rebuild new bone. When we are young and our bones are developing, osteoblasts work faster than osteoclasts, increasing bone density. Around age thirty, these two kinds of cells work at the same pace, maintaining bone density until roughly age fifty, at which time osteoclasts outpace osteoblasts and density decreases. If bones become too thin, then it is deemed osteoporosis.

I also learned that Phenobarbital, which I had been on as a child for temporal lobe seizures, was another risk factor; it interferes with calcium absorption. Dad was furious when I mentioned this to him. He doesn't recall the doctors covering that risk factor when discussing putting me on the medication. Dad said that had he known, he might have made a different decision, especially since I was taking the medication during my critical bone-forming years. Those are difficult decisions for parents to make for a child. Does one take a drug to fix an immediate problem, or does one refuse the drug in case it might cause another problem in the distant future? Furthermore, the risk of osteoporosis may not have even been known back then.

The month after I was diagnosed, Grandma fell and broke her hip. This was surprising as she still had quite strong bones; until the past couple of years, she walked everywhere. Her hugs were so strong that I thought she would crush me. I can remember Mom handing jars to Grandma, who opened them effortlessly. The surgeon commented that he really had to pound on the pin to get it into her hip when he operated. Unfortunately, her mind was not as strong as her bones; dementia had set in. Grandma never left the hospital. She died two months later.

Although I *knew* she had diabetes, dementia and high blood pressure, I *felt* that she died from a broken hip, which scared me. I was terrified of falling, which can happen any time with cp. I can do something a million times with no problem, and then fall the next time. If Grandma died two months after breaking her hip when her bones were still quite dense, how long would I have if I broke my hip? Grandma's doctor mentioned that approximately 25% of patients with broken hips do not recover and subsequently die. That did not alleviate my fear of falling.

I was very careful every time I moved from one seat to another or stood up. I made sure I always wore sturdy shoes so that a foot did not unexpectedly slip. I was vigilant about how much calcium I was eating. I took my Fosamax every Wednesday morning with plenty of water, as well as my daily calcium and vitamin D supplements. I envisioned my bones as micro construction sites with nano-sized bulldozers and front-end loaders building up my bones.

I also researched the kinds of exercises recommended to improve bone health. Walking was always listed as the number one exercise, which I found to be a rather circular statement. Had I been able to walk, I probably wouldn't have osteoporosis in the first place! Thus, walking was not a viable method for rectifying the situation. Through trial and error and listening to my body, I figured out what exercises I could do without aggravating my carpal tunnel and other aches and pains, and with a minimal gym in our home.

What felt like a shin splint kept coming and going that summer. I didn't really pay attention until early fall when I noticed the pain seemed to return Thursday or Friday, and then dissipated by Monday. Other unexplainable bone-stabbing pains began occurring. Was I experiencing growing pains at age thirty-something? If my bones were becoming denser and healthier, this made sense. But the pain was intensifying as the weeks passed. By November, I was doubled over in pain on Thursday or Friday. Then the pain would be gone by Monday, only to return by Thursday. Could it be the Fosamax that I was taking Wednesday morning?

During that time, I was feeling somewhat depressed. I thought perhaps Grandma's death had hit me unexpectedly hard. She was my last living grandparent and the only one I knew well. My other grandparents had died when I was fairly young. I don't remember Grandpa Watson at all, and I vaguely remember Papa and Nana Marshall. With Grandma now gone, it meant my parents were now next in line to *get old* and then to pass away, a rather unsettling and uncomforting thought. I can't imagine being without my parents. Despite the miles that separate us right now, they are always there for me. I know that if I ever really needed something, they will both be here as soon as possible. I can't and don't want to imagine them not in my life.

The end of November, I went to my family doctor for my flu shot. I also went with a list of typed questions in hand, including one about Fosamax possibly causing the bone pain. The doctor's response was that bones don't have pain, so Fosamax couldn't possibly be causing the pain. He offered the explanation that I was likely experiencing deep muscle tightness due to my cp. Because of my unclear speech, I held back on saying, *No, I've had cp all my life, and this is a new pain that occurs the day after my weekly dose of Fosamax.* I also refrained from explaining that I had read the full drug monograph online and that it says, in a few cases, patients experience joint and bone pain. In rare cases, malaise has been reported. Hmm, isn't malaise a synonym for depression? Maybe I wasn't losing it after all. I left the doctor's office, feeling unheard and unacknowledged as an intelligent woman who knows and understands her own body.

I continued being a compliant patient until sometime in January when I was so doubled over in pain and dreading Wednesday mornings that Darrell called the doctor to explain the situation again. The doctor again tried to contribute the pain to my cp, but Darrell emphatically explained that this was a new pain occurring every Thursday, after taking Fosamax on Wednesday. The doctor said he had no other patient complain about Fosamax. Who cares? I'm not the same as every other patient! Perhaps he didn't hear them either when they did complain. He finally relented and told Darrell that the only way to know for sure was to stop taking Fosamax for one month. Well, it didn't take a month for the pain to disappear. It stopped immediately! And I have yet to experience that sharp, bone-stabbing pain again! The fog also lifted and colour came back into my life. I was able to focus more and to get things accomplished. I was Glenda again.

In my research, I discovered there was a multi-disciplinary Osteoporosis Clinic at the Women's Health Centre, located within BC Women's Hospital (formerly Grace Hospital, where I was born). I reluctantly visit the Centre's Access Clinic for my annual thrill as it has one of the very few accessible exam tables in the province. Obviously, the sexual health of women with disabilities is not a priority to the Ministry of Health! Rather than going through my family doctor for the requisite referral, I contacted the gynecologist. Once I finally had an appointment after a lengthy wait, I met with the nutritionist, the specialist and the clinic nurse all in one day – the physio was away that day. It was great to be able to ask questions and to have them answered in a non-condescending way. From my experience so far, the Centre's doctors and nurses readily acknowledge that knowledge is power, and they aren't averse to sharing information with the patient, even if the patient has a disability! I find that a refreshing and much welcomed concept.

Meeting with the specialist, she confirmed my experience with Fosamax; sometimes it can cause bone pain. She was surprised that my doctor hadn't believed me. She wanted to try another medication, but, acknowledging my reluctance to something else and my preference to try a calcium-rich diet and exercise, she agreed to wait until my next bone density scan. If there was a decrease or no improvement, she would strongly recommend that I try another drug. That bone scan and a subsequent one have shown marked improvements. I am drug-free, and my goal is to remain that way!

Christmas 2005, I was setting the table for dinner. I was either rushing a little too much as company was due shortly or I wasn't as careful as I should have been. As I reached to put a fork in place, I felt myself go beyond my point of balance. I let out an "I know what is coming next but there is nothing I can do about it" groan as I fell in slow motion to the floor. We should have gone with softwood floors!

Dad was spending Christmas with us, and he came running from Darrell's office where he was doing some last minute gift-wrapping. Putting his first aid ticket to use, he had me lay still for a bit until everything stopped reverberating. He then slowly eased me up and back onto my scooter. Nothing was broken!

In that moment I realized that I could fall without breaking anything, without dying. It was such a relief! Not that I want to make it a frequent occurrence. It means I don't need to be so terrified about it. That fear is no longer always in the back of my mind. I think being careful and vigilant is one thing, but always being in fear is not really living; it's avoiding death. And that is no way live life to its fullest.

COMING OUT OF THE SILENCE

Despite my inability to walk without falling every few steps, which doesn't tend to get me very far, very fast, and my limited hand function, my unclear speech is my biggest frustration. One of the guidance counsellors in high school asked me if I would prefer to be able to walk or to talk. Definitely talk! I have lived a fairly full life, even though I have done most of it from a wheelchair. I don't feel I have missed out on *too* much, and I definitely don't understand the looks of pity I get from strangers when they see me in my scooter. At least I am guaranteed a seat everywhere I go!

But my speech is a different story. The finger spelling and alphanumeric calculator I used in Brownies and Guides, the notes I typed to high school teachers, the *talking papers* I used all through university, the alphabet card I wouldn't leave home without, and the postcard business spiels all allowed for limited interaction with others. However, none were as natural or as liberating as clear speech, something most people take for granted and don't stop to appreciate. Being "functioning non-verbal", as labelled by the medical experts, has led to isolation and loneliness at times. Without clear speech, simple interactions with other people are difficult. And when people do hear my speech, they mistakenly assume I am deaf or cognitively impaired, neither of which could be further from the truth.

Shortly after Darrell and I moved in together, the supervisor from the homemaking agency came to assess us for services. She essentially asked the same questions as the Long-Term Care case manager had asked a couple of weeks earlier. She also examined our bathroom. I think these people must have a bathroom fetish as they all insist on seeing it. Forget any sense of privacy when you have a disability.

As she began the interview process, she turned to me and said, "You aren't very articulate. I'm going to speak with him," pointing to Darrell, the verbal one. Handing me a brochure, she continued, "Here, you can look at this. Can you read?" Feeling totally insulted and disregarded, I so much wanted to kick her out of my home! But, afraid that she might note *uncooperative, bitter client* on the file, as many people with disabilities get labelled, I bit my tongue and swallowed the insult and hurt once again. As if that wasn't bad enough, she added, "I used to work with people like you. I understand." Sarcastically, I thought, *You must have been great at that job, too!*

Once she left, I immediately wrote a letter to her supervisor, detailing what her employee had said to me in my own home. I neither heard back, nor received an apology. This was yet another unenlightened soul that entered my life ever so briefly, but her words remain with me.

Other times, particularly in groups, I can feel so totally alone. I remember being at one conference, in a roomful of approximately 400 people, and I felt immensely alone and invisible. Ironically, the conference was for employers eager to "do the right thing" by hiring people with disabilities! I thought they would make the effort to get to know me to enhance their knowledge and understanding of people with disabilities or possibly to offer me a job, but it didn't happen.

Along the way, people with good intentions have suggested that I try various communication devices. But, being the stubborn one that I am – to which Darrell can attest – I graciously refused. Long before Microsoft and its Speech Application Programming Interface or SAPI, I felt the early speech synthesizers were more difficult to understand than I was. I opted to stick with my typed notes, my alphabet card and my silence.

The internet has opened a whole new world to me. I can finally communicate with others without my disability getting in the way. Oftentimes, others don't even know I have a disability. If they do, they don't know the extent of it. This means we can have more meaningful exchanges because we can bypass the misperceptions and misunderstandings of my cerebral palsy and get right to the topic at hand. It is such a liberating feeling! And, it is amazing who all I have connected with online.

Email, online conferences and discussion forums enable me to participate fully in the virtual world and to lead the exciting life of an online solopreneur. Although this technology means greater inclusion in participating in the virtual world, there is a risk of becoming further isolated from the real world. The very technology tools that allow me to be accepted into the world as an equal can also isolate me even more as I draw further and further into the "virtual world" with less and less "real life", face-to-face contact with human beings.

In April 2005, I temporarily escaped *Hermitsville* when I was asked to speak at the Social Planning and Research Council of British Columbia's (SPARC BC), "Beyond the Obvious: Exploring the Accessible Community Dialogue".

My initial thought was *But I don't give speeches. I can't.* Since I was raised without the word *"can't "*in my vocabulary, that was a fleeing thought. I quickly turned my thought to *How can I do this?*

I had been using the free computer software ReadPlease for a couple of years to proofread my writing. ReadPlease reads aloud text that is copied into the program. I thought, *Maybe I could put ReadPlease onto my laptop and have it read aloud my speech for me.* I hesitantly agreed to speak. Unsure if the technology would work, I took a printed copy of the speech with me, in case I needed someone else to read it on my behalf.

Finally, it was my turn to take the stage. Being on stage alone for the first time in my life, with two hundred eyes staring at me, I wanted to run. But, I didn't. I gave my speech. When I was done, I left the stage, trembling. I had given my first ever speech! And the technology worked!

Afterwards something amazing happened. For the rest of the day people actually came up to me and spoke with me. I was heard for the first time. I was no longer invisible, no longer silent. It was an amazing, unexplainable feeling that I would like to experience again. I would like to give more speeches. I would like to be heard again.

A few weeks prior to writing this, the World Urban Forum, a United Nations event, was held here in beautiful Vancouver, British Columbia. I attended the session on accessibility and inclusion conducted by SPARC BC, of which I am now on the Board of Directors thanks to that first speech! Because I had participated in the practice run of the event a week or so earlier, I was able to prepare some comments for the live event.

Using a text-to-mp3 converter and a newly acquired synthesized voice, Kate by NeoSpeech, I was able to convert my written word into spoken word and then play the file on my laptop at the appropriate time! The voice isn't mine; but I don't use my own legs for mobility either, yet I can still get around. Actually, when I first heard Kate, I jumped out of my chair! She was so clear, for a computer, and perhaps even somewhat sexy! It was love at the first sound byte.

Using my synthesized voice on my laptop and my pre-canned comments, I actually put up my hand to *say* something for the first time in my life! Again, people came up to me afterwards to say they liked what I had said. I was invited to another event in July because of what I had said. It's like by becoming *verbal*, I become *visible, too*. To be completely honest, I am hungry to do more.

Using this same text-to-mp3 technology, now I can even podcast! This non-verbal red-head is podcasting! I feel like a butterfly, emerging from my cocoon of silence. I can now reach people in a new way, and who knows what opportunities will arise now that I can podcast!

I no longer consider myself non-verbal; instead, I have a significant speech impairment. This has been an empowering experience as I try on words that better describe and define me, rather than being burden with labels imposed upon me by medical professionals or strangers. It will continue to be a journey, a process, as I transition from being non-verbal to speech impaired. This will likely mean taking steps, even baby steps, as I take on this new role. I still need to find a way to have spontaneous dialogue, something more than pre-canned utterances. I also need to build up my confidence in communicating in this way. But with Darrell's encouragement and support, we will continue creatively experimenting with technology until we find solutions that work for me. Soon, I'll be ready for Oprah and Larry King!

To be continued....

EPILOGUE

In writing this book, I was selective in what memories to include in this written photo album. This means that some friends, relatives and acquaintances were not mentioned within these pages. Please do not feel slighted in the least if you are one of them.

I appreciate and value all those who have come into my life as friends; those who were able to see beyond the cp to see me; those who have taken the time to learn *Glenda-ish* to get to know the real me. It is you who have made life easier for me.

In a world where accessibility is still a struggle, it is people's attitudes and acceptance that make all the difference. That is what can make my day a great day! And for those who took the time to make my day great, I am sincerely grateful.

Two people I am especially grateful for are my parents. They believed in me since Day One, when some doctors – the "experts" – said that I should be institutionalized and forgotten, that I would not amount to anything. My parents encouraged me, telling me that I could do anything that I put my mind to. They told me there was no such word as *can't;* only *try*, and to always try my best. They taught me to always say "Thank you," and that if the words wouldn't clearly come in that moment, then to smile – a smile CAN open doors.

They spent hours beside my hospital bed; Mom knitting as I tried to sleep despite the pain and Dad using a straw to drop juice into my mouth so that I didn't have to move, and thus, avoiding more pain. No doubt it was as heartbreaking for them when they had to leave as it was for me when they left at the end of visiting hours. There were tears on both sides of the door.

They were always supportive no matter what I wanted to try, whether it was going to Brownies, starting horseback riding, leaving for university, getting married or buying a condo. Putting their own personal pain aside, they were both there for my convocation, my wedding and my fortieth birthday, which meant a lot to me. And now, despite them having been divorced for several years, they still offer the exact same words of advice and encouragement.

So, now, in front of all those who took the time to read these ramblings, for which I am thankful, I would like to thank my parents for believing in me, for encouraging me and for supporting me. You have helped me to reach my dreams and to become the woman who I am today. Thank you, Mom and Dad. I love you.